About the author

Claire Oxenham was born and raised in Cheshire, England and moved to Australia 14 years ago. She lives a (somewhat) quiet life with her husband and three young boys.

This Isn't Eczema is a personal project that draws on Claire's own visceral 15-month battle with topical steroid withdrawal (TSW).

Her motivation for writing the book was to give those experiencing or facing TSW hope, advice and a chuckle of recognition.

Ultimately, it's a guidebook, a symbol of solidarity, and a means of raising awareness about this 'rare' condition.

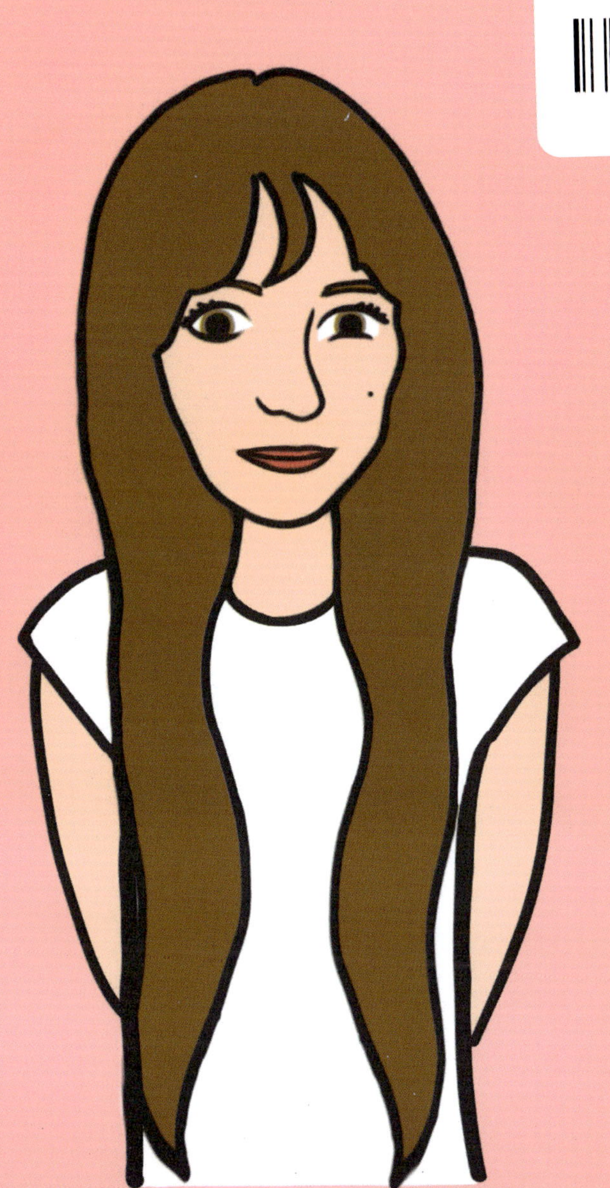

About the Illustrator

Charlotte Oxenham is a talented artist from the UK. She skilfully captures emotion and likeness in any subject, using a variety of techniques.

Her works draw from personal experiences, such as anxiety and insecurity, which perfectly aligns with the themes in this book.

View more of Charlotte's work:

charlotteoxenhamart.com

@artby_charl

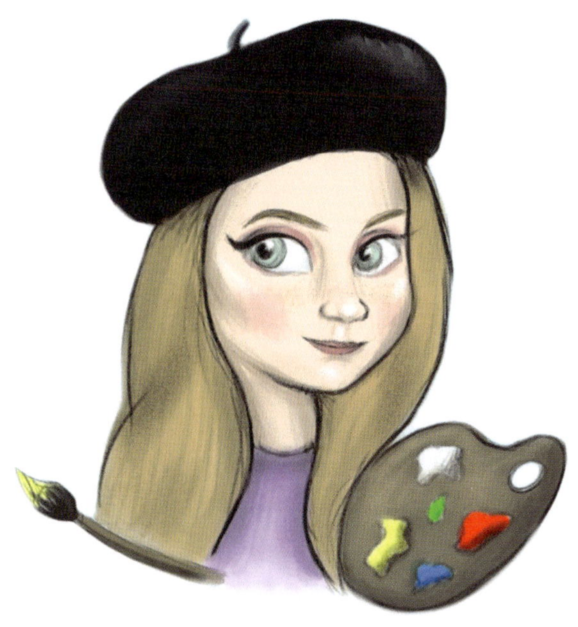

Title: **This Isn't Eczema**
What to expect when you're going through topical steroid withdrawal

First Edition

Published by Little ARO May 2021

A R O

Text by Claire Oxenham

Illustrations © by Charlotte Oxenham

EBOOK ISBN: 978-0-6451411-0-8

PB ISBN: 978-0-6451411-1-5

THIS ISN'T ECZEMA

What to Expect When You're Going Through
Topical Steroid Withdrawal

CLAIRE OXENHAM
Illustrations by CHARLOTTE OXENHAM

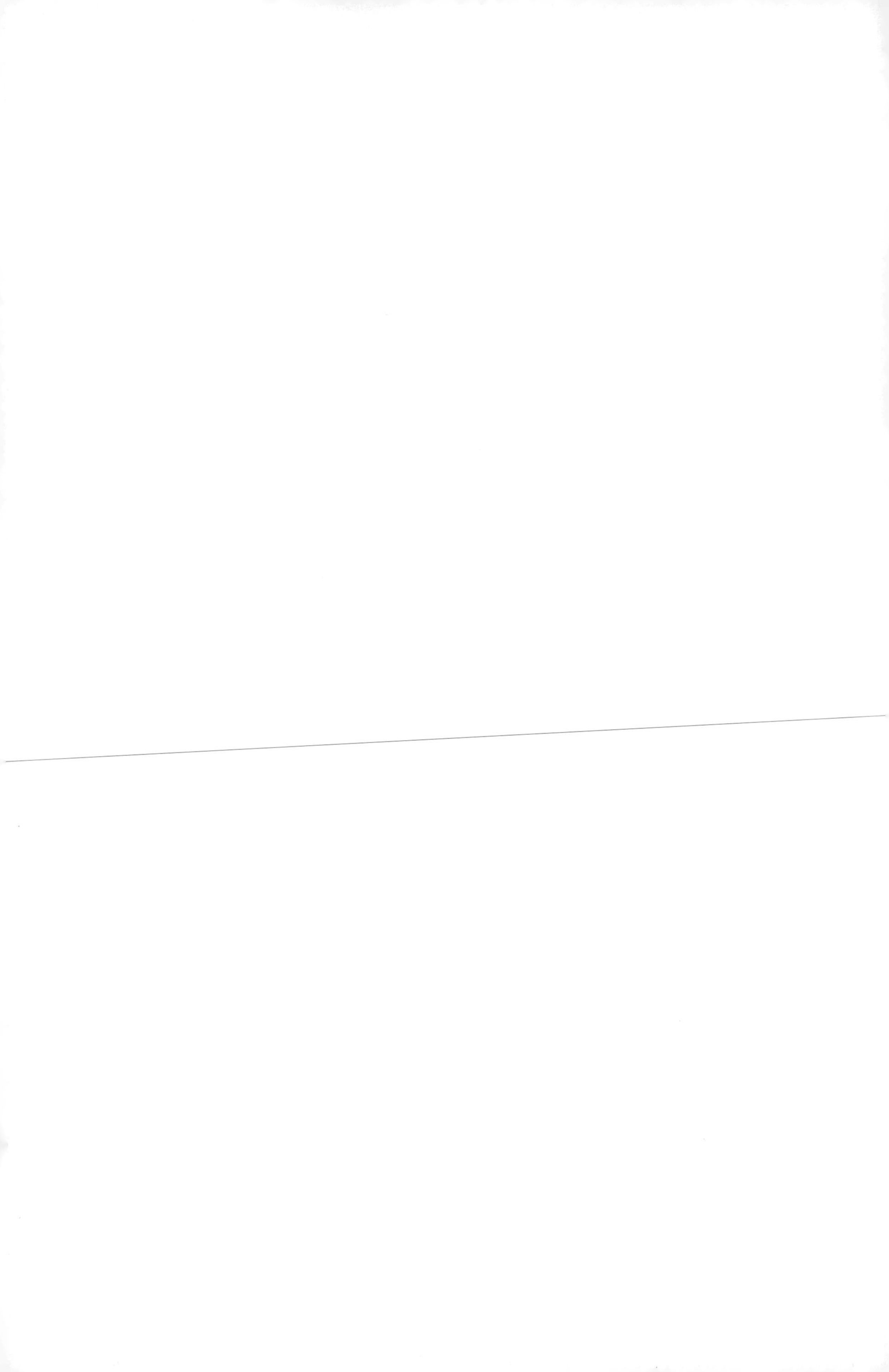

Disclaimer

I must make it clear that I'm not a medical professional, neither have I studied TSW or gained qualifications in dermatology or related fields. I have, however, lived through TSW. This qualifies me to discuss the condition from direct first-hand experience. I've also carried out heavy independent research over 15 months as part of the TSW community.

This book isn't meant to be used and shouldn't be used to diagnose or treat any medical condition, neither has it been approved by a regulating body. Readers should consult with their doctor if TSW is suspected.

Laughter through the pain

Although this book has some fun pictures and light-hearted comments, I can't stress the seriousness of TSW enough.

It can be hell on earth and affect you so severely, both physically and mentally, that you think you can't go on. When you feel this way, know that you can. Our community will hold your hand and guide and support you at every stage.

The advice, words, descriptions, expectations, and symptoms I've listed here draw on my own experiences and those of other members of the TSW community.

If you suffer with TSW, you may experience all the symptoms I've listed or just a handful. Everyone has their own unique journey, and I sincerely hope you don't suffer too much.

For my boys

Thank you for putting up with my constant scratching

For the TSW community

With love

Why I wrote this book

'Do you want the answer? Or do you want *the answer*?'

The skin specialist was looking at me dead in the eye, eager to give his opinion.

I'd just spent the past 20 minutes telling him about my symptoms and how I'd been going through hell ever since I stopped using topical steroid medication.

He'd assessed me in full, taking his time, looking at every square inch of my body– my angry red burning skin, my swollen lymph nodes, my flaking areas, and my wrinkled legs and arms. These were just some of the many symptoms I'd shown or explained to him.

He was a local doctor specialising in skin I'd sought out for a professional opinion, and I was struck by how confident he was and his promise of holding 'the answer'.

The answer he gave me was this: 'You have severe chronic eczema and will need to be on steroid medication, probably ongoing, for the rest of your life.'

Wow.

This was what he was so sure of?

This was *'the answer'*?

Luckily for me, I'd spent the past few months researching topical steroid withdrawal (TSW), and I knew that what I had wasn't eczema at all. The condition I had was actually the result of using eczema medication.

But what if I hadn't been researching it? What if I didn't know TSW existed? What if I just followed his advice to continue using topical steroids at a stronger dose for years to come? What if I was a parent doing this to my child?

This was the moment I decided to dedicate every spare minute I had to raising awareness about this condition.

This was the catalyst for the book.

My story from the beginning

I suffered from mild eczema on my arm as a child and was prescribed the first-line treatment: topical steroid cream. I used this infrequently for a few years, and, over time, my skin slowly became worse, leading to a diagnosis of moderate eczema.

After consistent treatment, year after year, with increasingly stronger topical steroids, I'd started to develop what was fast becoming an unmanageable skin condition. I decided enough was enough. By then, my skin had stopped responding to the creams, and with burning red skin, I was finding no relief.

A lifetime on topical and oral steroids was not feasible for me. It didn't seem right that that was the only option, so I spent hours researching the cause of my red skin and stumbled across some blogs discussing TSW. I couldn't believe it; the symptoms were identical to mine. It was my lightbulb moment. I realised my skin had become addicted to the steroids and that I needed to go through it.

Going against the grain, I stopped using steroids and entered full-body withdrawal. This withdrawal lasted 15 months and was, at times, absolutely brutal. It was immense and all-consuming.

I went into withdrawal against the advice of every medical specialist I saw. All consistently told me that it was just 'worsening eczema'. I knew it wasn't. I'd come to realise that my medication wasn't getting stronger because my skin was getting worse. My skin was getting worse because my medication had been getting stronger.

So I withdrew from topical and oral steroids with no medication, no creams, and no products. I just allowed my body to heal naturally.

I'm now at a stage where the worst of my symptoms have subsided, and I'm absolutely committed to raising awareness and educating people about the dangers of topical steroids and their unintentional over-use from over-prescription.

This book is for people wondering why their 'eczema' is getting worse but who have no answers.

It's for people just starting their journey into TSW and finding it all a bit overwhelming and confusing.

It's to raise awareness about the condition and to continue expanding our conversations about the effects of topical steroids.

And it's also to make you smile, even in your darkest TSW days.

Understanding topical steroids and TSW

What are topical steroids?

Topical steroid creams are a synthetic (man-made) corticosteroid medication used for treating a **variety of skin conditions**.

Why are topical steroids used?

Topical steroids are medications of varying strength used to **reduce inflammation and itching**.

They're commonly used to treat rashes, eczema, dermatitis and psoriasis. They're also used for sunburn, heat rash, nappy rash, shaving rash, bites and stings. Some require a prescription; others are available over-the-counter or at the pharmacy. You might also see topical steroids being sold as miracle 'cure-all' creams online.

How do topical steroids work?

Topical steroids mimic the body's natural hormones, which our adrenal glands would usually produce.

The steroids suppress inflammation that occurs when our skin has an allergic reaction or stress response. They constrict the blood vessels, reducing redness.

They can seem wondrously effective – a miracle cure. However, the reality is that **they only hide the cause of the redness; they don't treat it**.

It's important to understand that topical steroids affect our body in a very complex way. It's not just the specific area of the skin's surface that's affected. Topical steroids are also absorbed into our skin and bloodstream. Because of this, they can affect the body's immune system, endocrine system and blood vessels.

Topical steroid addiction

It can take only a few weeks for the body to become dependent on topical steroids.

A tolerance to the medication can develop, resulting in the need for stronger prescribed drugs, with a clear rebound effect upon withdrawal.

Unfortunately, topical steroids are often prescribed for months or years, with the rebound symptoms often being diagnosed as a **'worsening eczema'**.

It can take days, weeks or months for the drug to leave your system completely, so symptoms can occur at different times. Many factors come in to play, including the level of potency, type of medication, frequency of use, age, areas of skin applied (all body parts absorb the cream at different rates), condition and thickness of the skin.

What is topical steroid withdrawal?

Topical steroid withdrawal (TSW) is a **type of drug withdrawal**.

It's a condition experienced by people who stop using topical steroids. Some TSW symptoms can appear while topical steroids are still being used. This is because the body becomes tolerant. It can take many months, or more commonly, many years, for someone to recover from TSW.

When you stop using topical steroids, withdrawal becomes all-encompassing. The entire body can be affected, not just the area where the steroids were used.

It's important to note that not everyone who uses topical steroid creams will get TSW. But for those who do, it can be devastating.

TSW has many symptoms – symptoms I've outlined in this book so that you know what to expect based on my own experience.

Advanced TSW looks very different to regular eczema because of the range of symptoms experienced. However, the early stages of TSW can look a lot like eczema. This is why it's often misdiagnosed early on.

Curing TSW

There are options available to alleviate mental and physical pain during withdrawal and to help manage infections.

There is, however, no cure for TSW. The body has to withdraw and recover.

The best course of action is prevention. This is why research, education and awareness are so important.

Some people may find certain therapies and medications helpful and comforting during withdrawal. Everyone's journey is different.

A note on terminology

Topical steroid withdrawal (TSW) is the term most frequently used. However, the condition is also referred to as **topical steroid addiction** (TSA) and **red skin syndrome** (RSS).

While I refer to topical steroid creams, withdrawal symptoms have also been reported by people after using oral steroids or steroid ointments, lotions or gels.

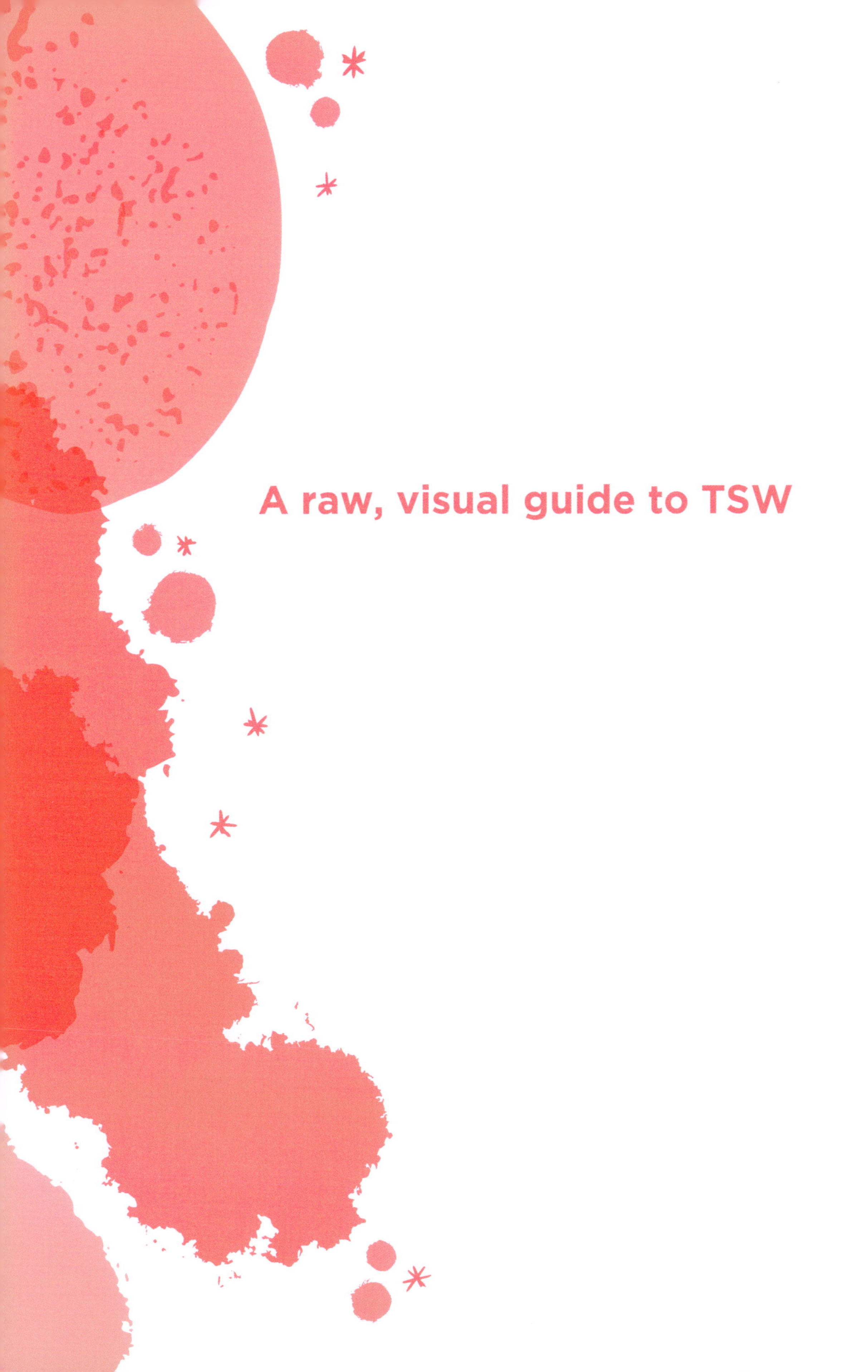

A raw, visual guide to TSW

You'll have painful burning skin.

It will feel like you're on fire.

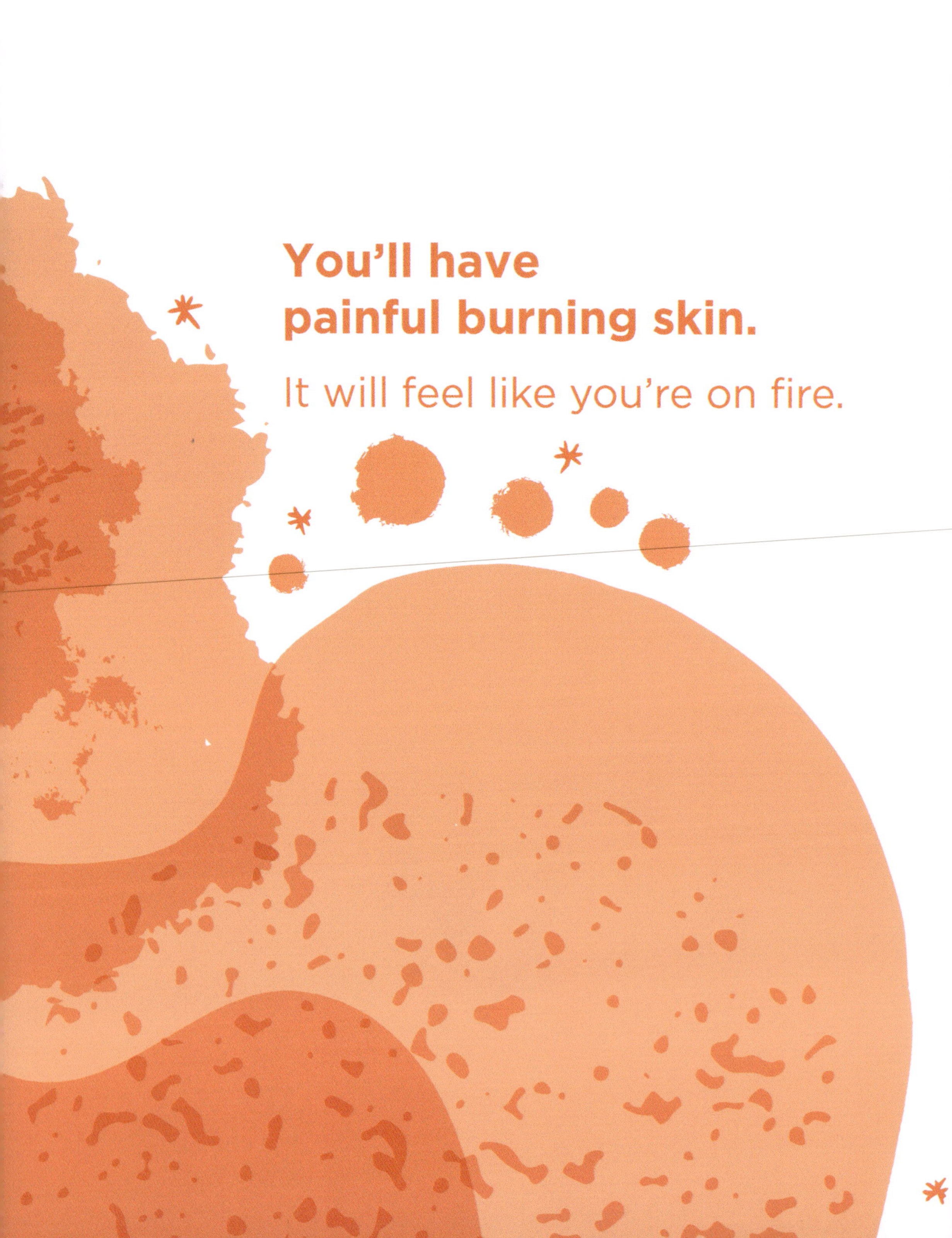

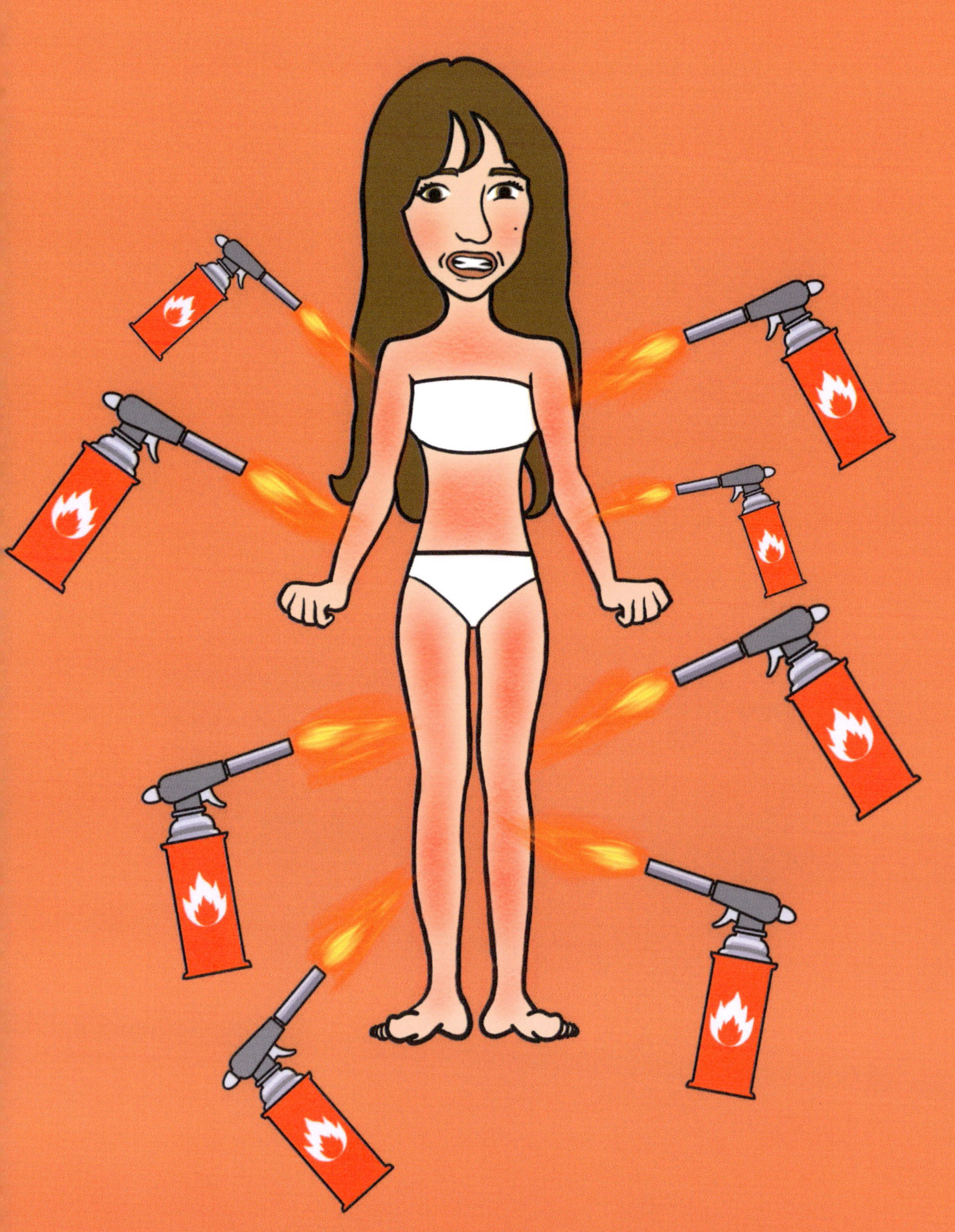

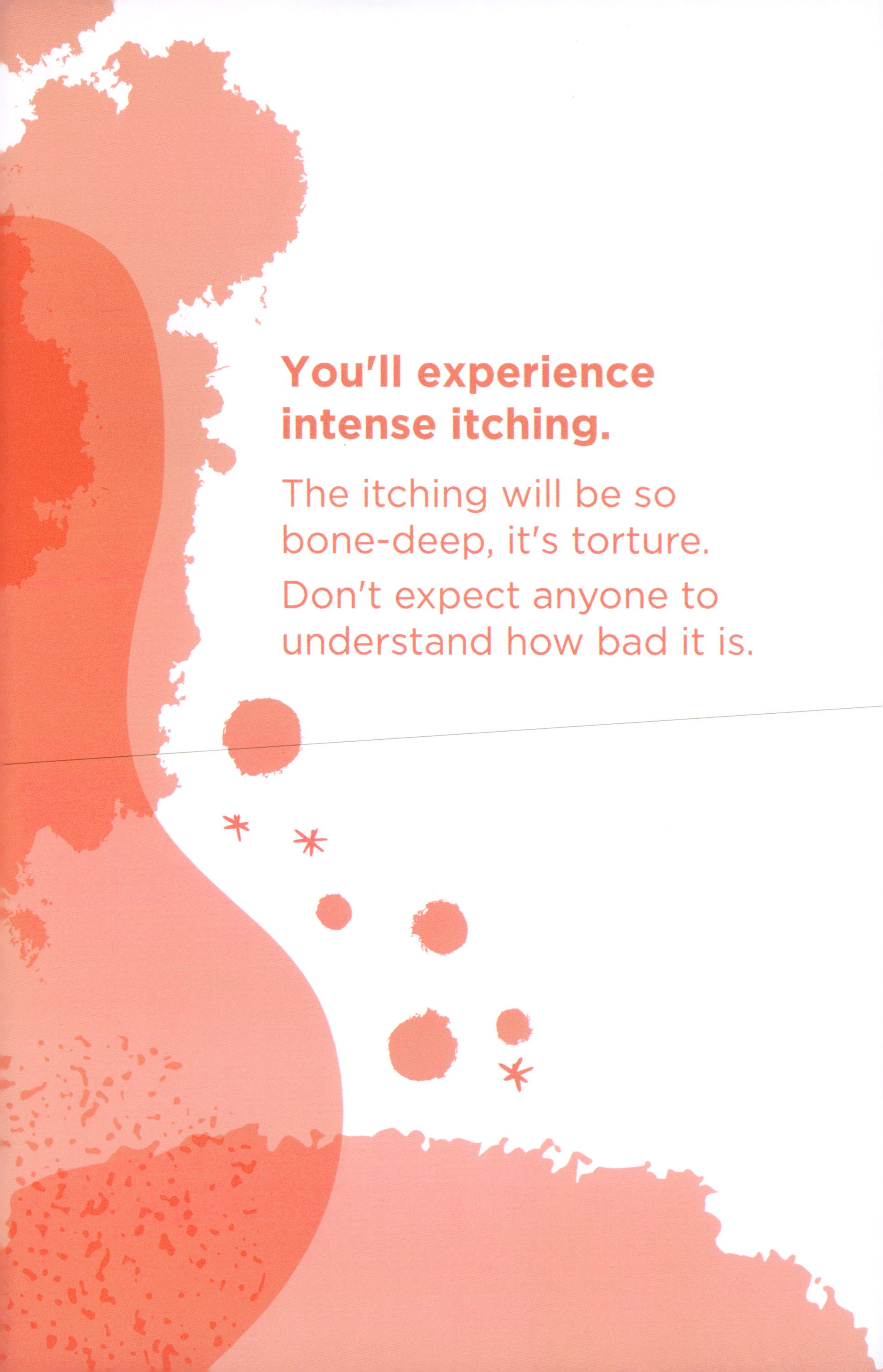

You'll experience intense itching.

The itching will be so bone-deep, it's torture.

Don't expect anyone to understand how bad it is.

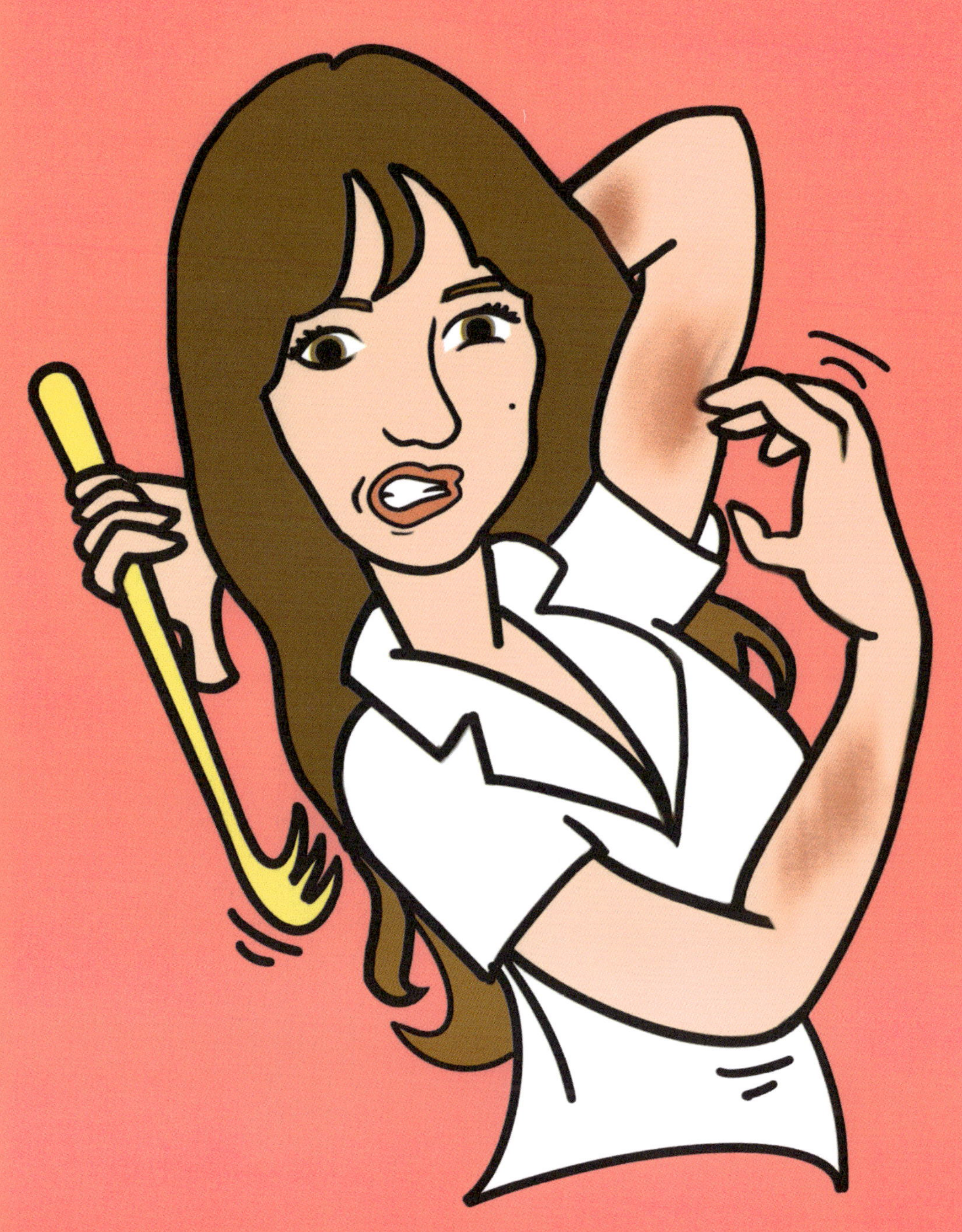

Skin flakes will be endless.

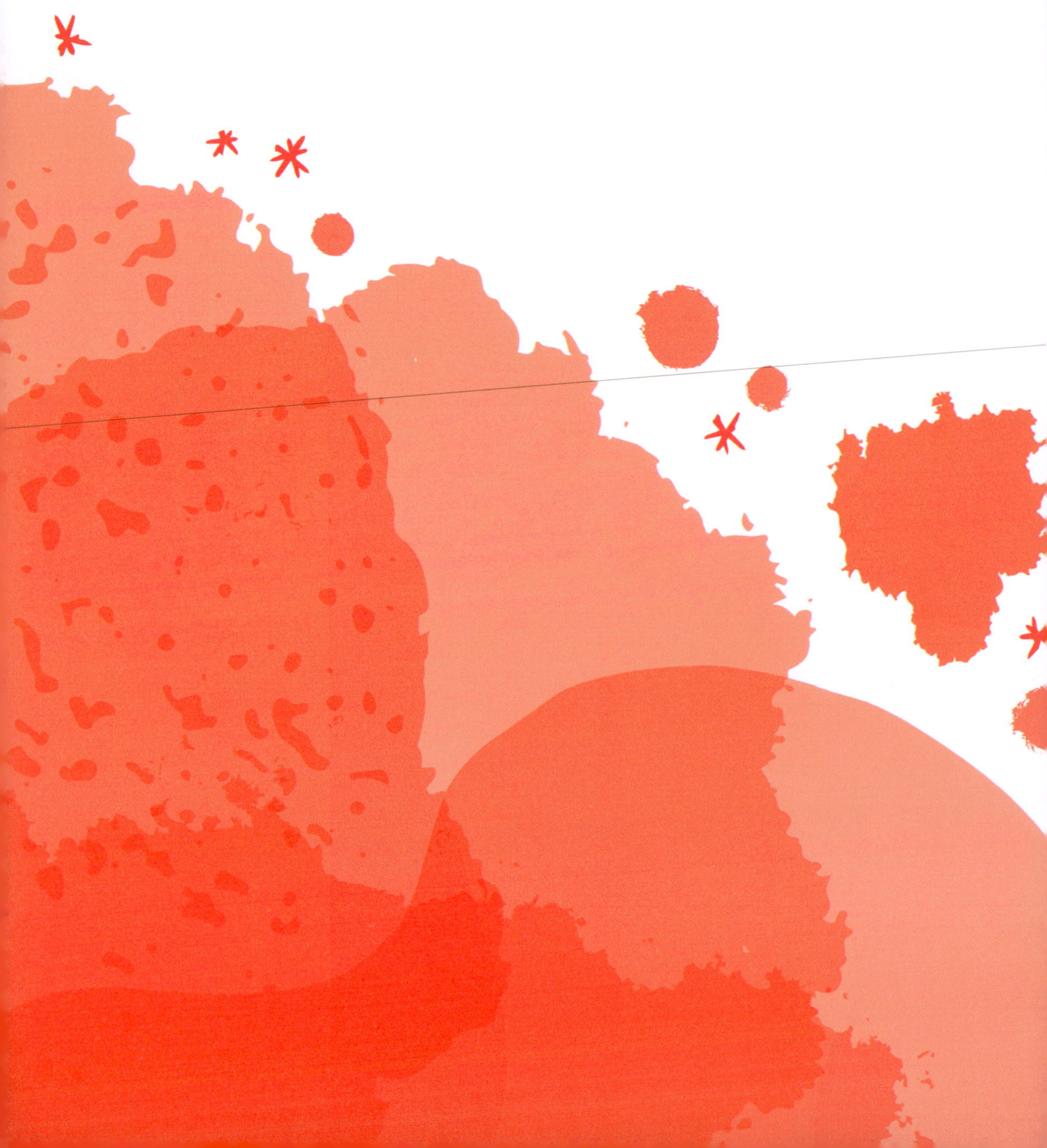

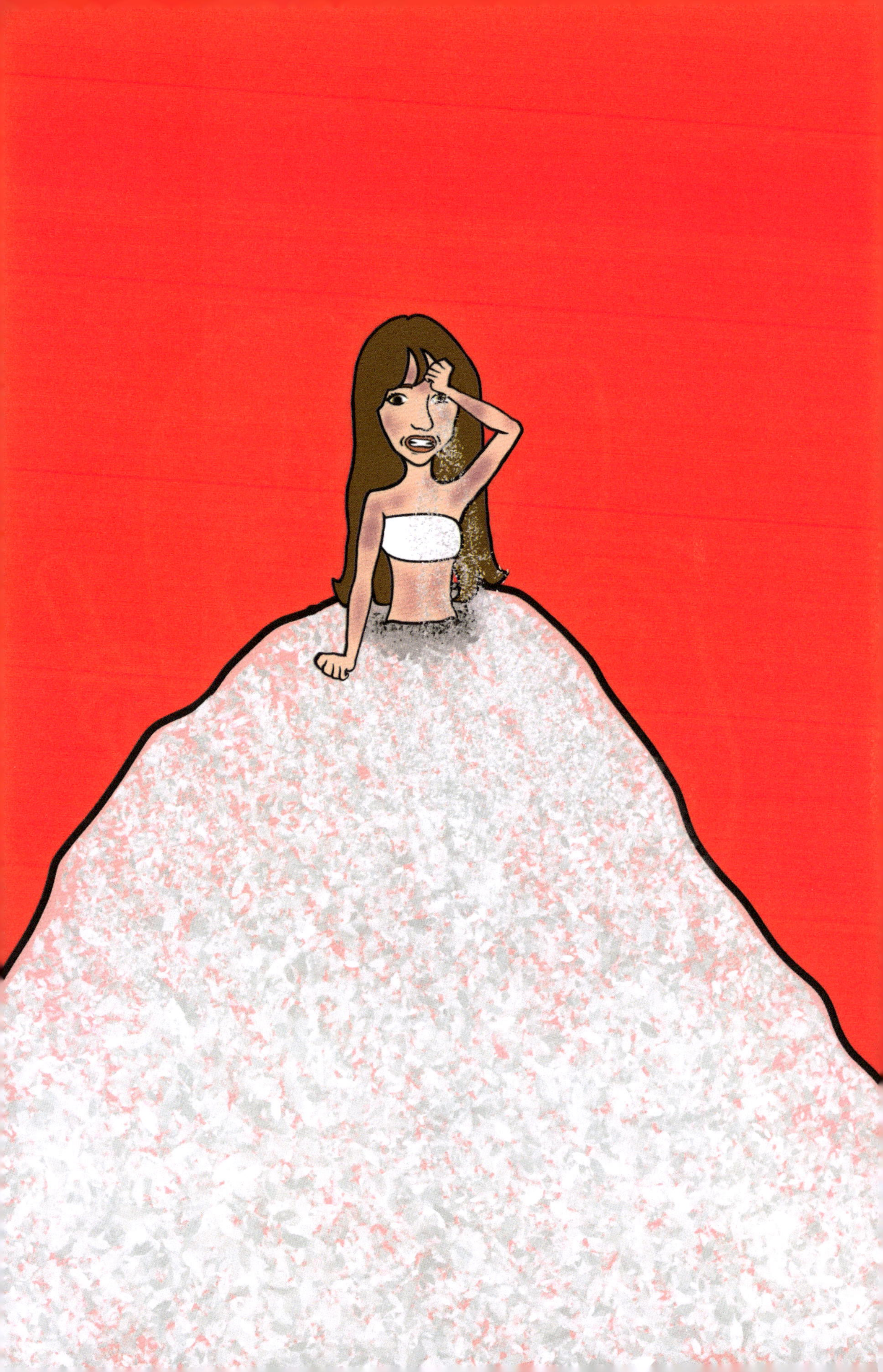

Face flakes can get quite scary.

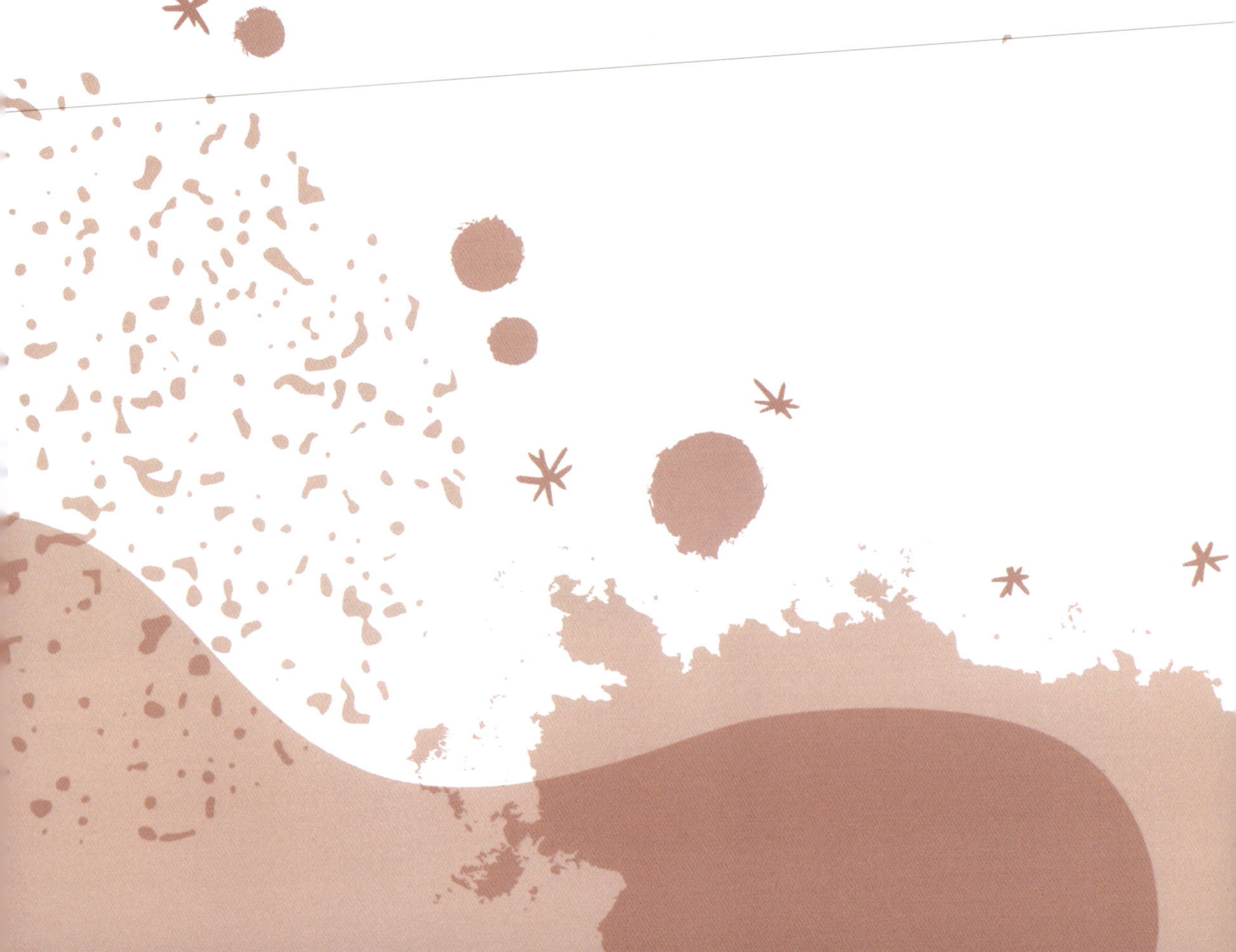

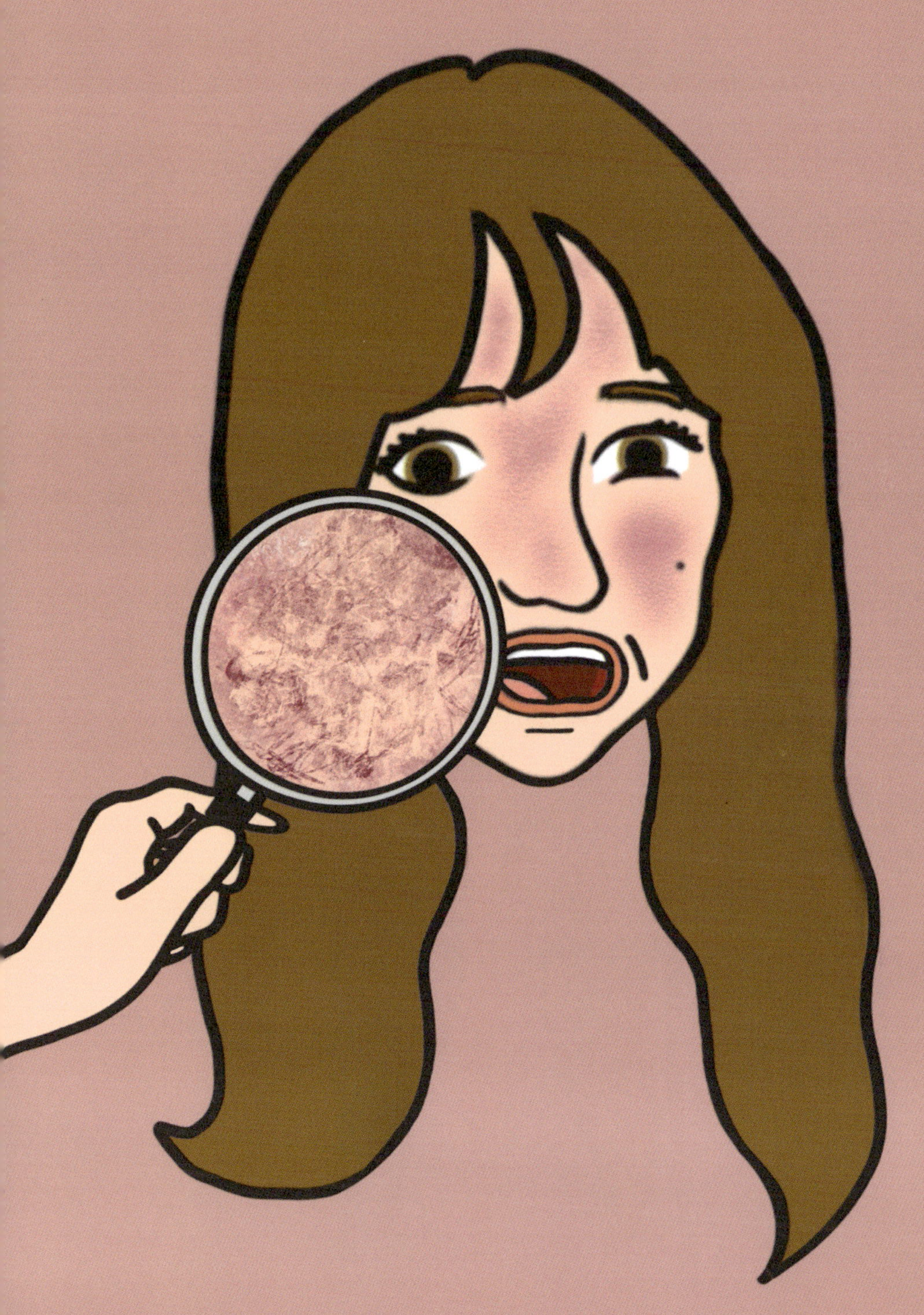

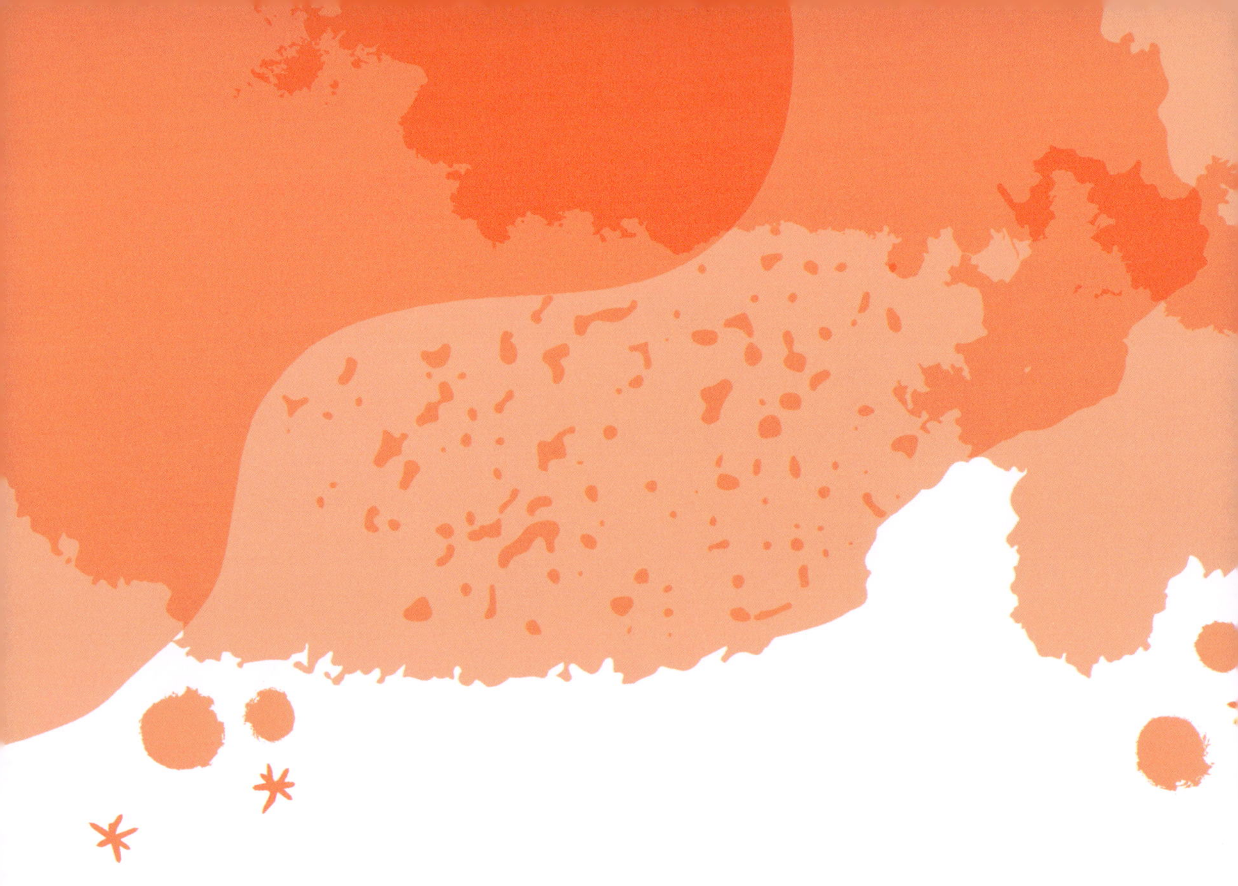

You'll purchase new products.

You'll buy so many things
in the hope of easing your pain.

But nothing works.

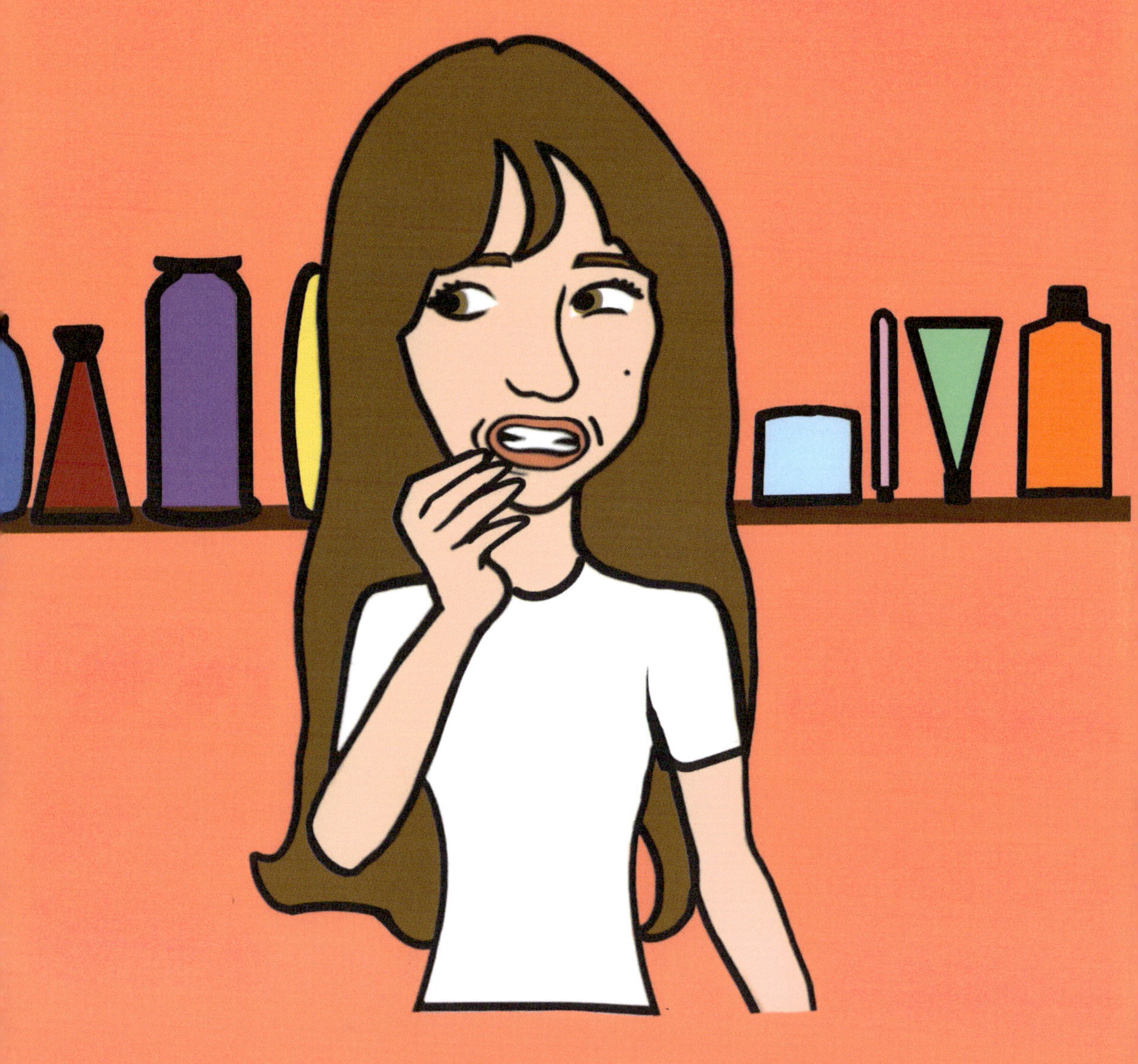

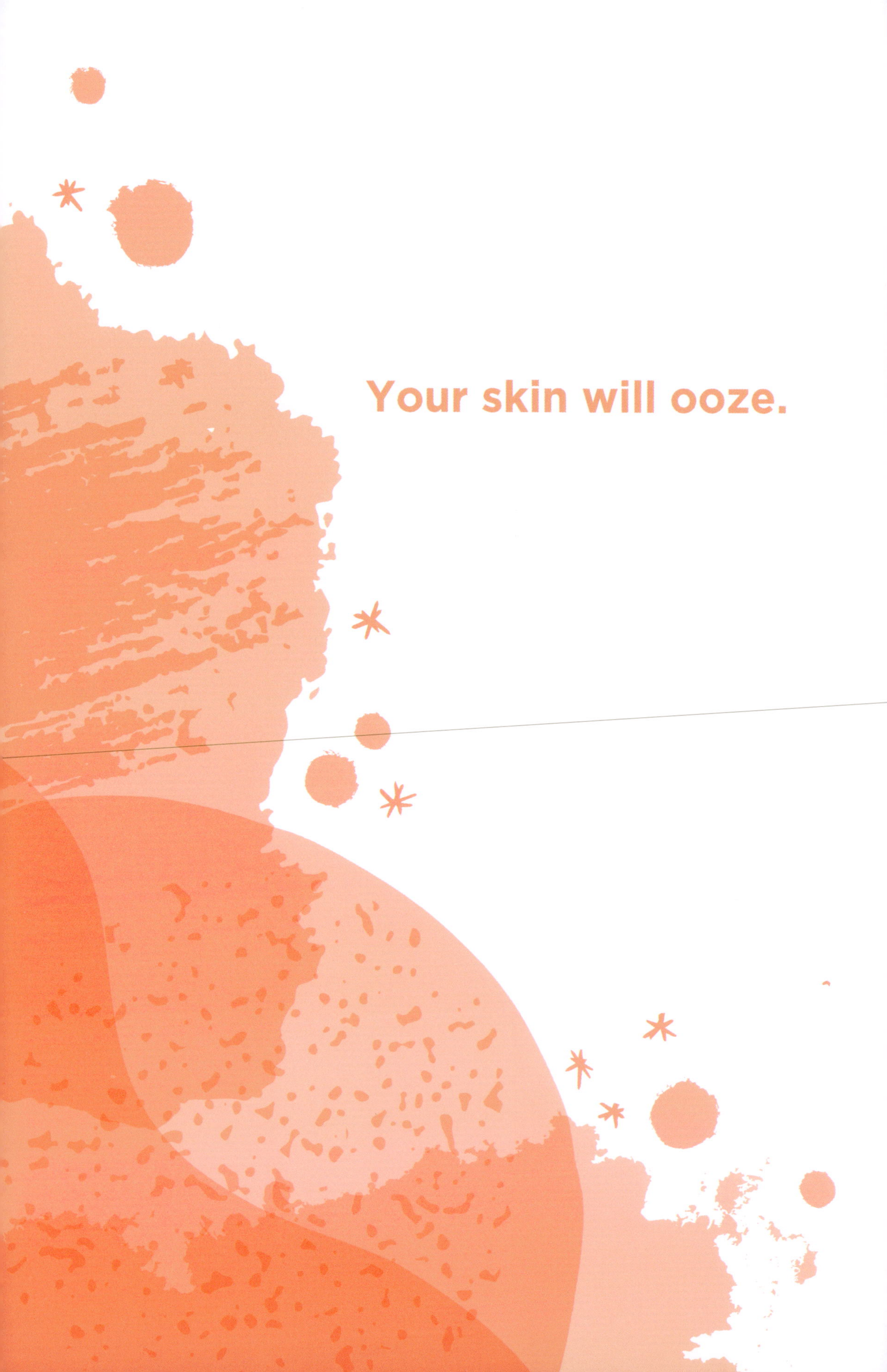

Your skin will ooze.

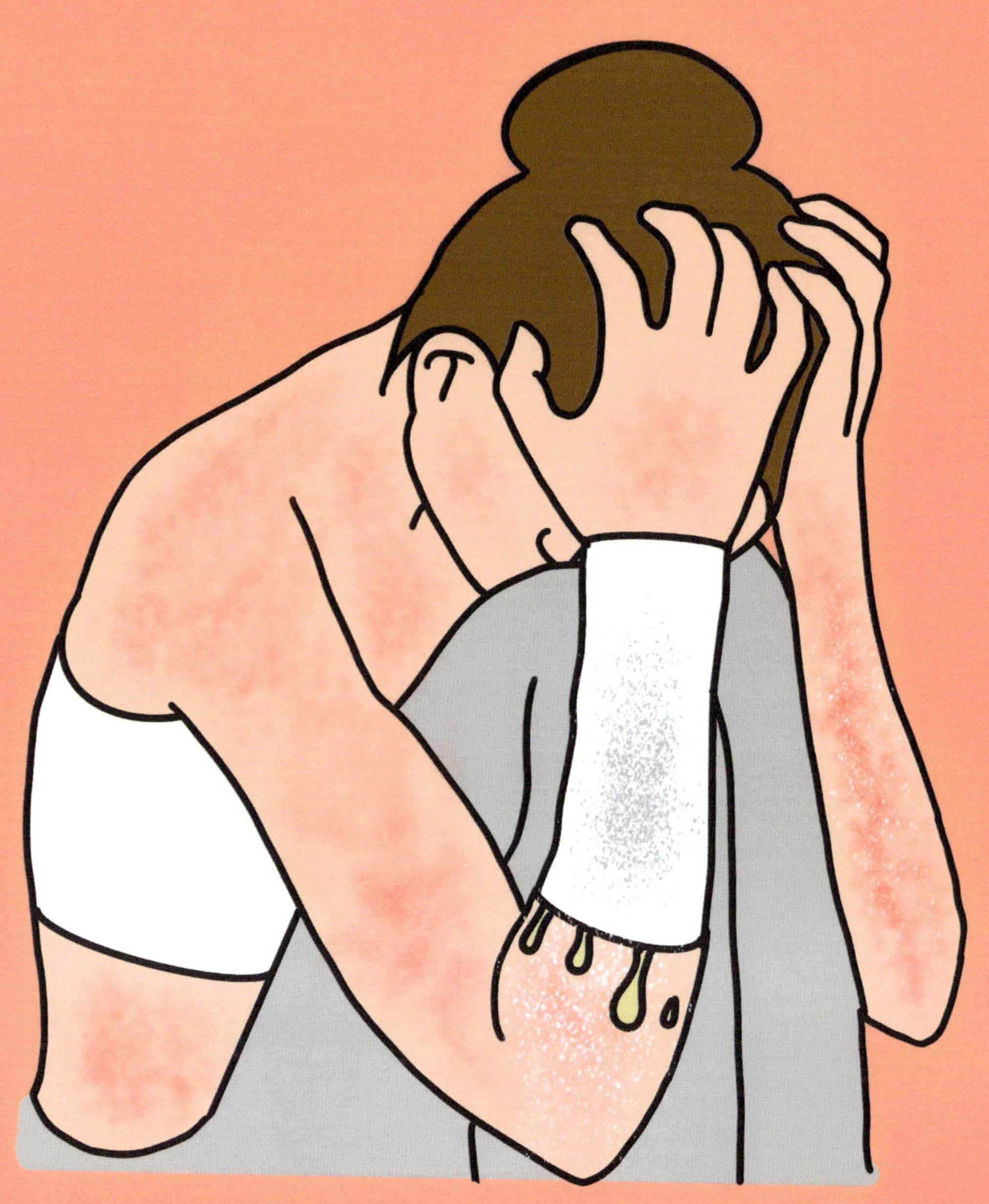

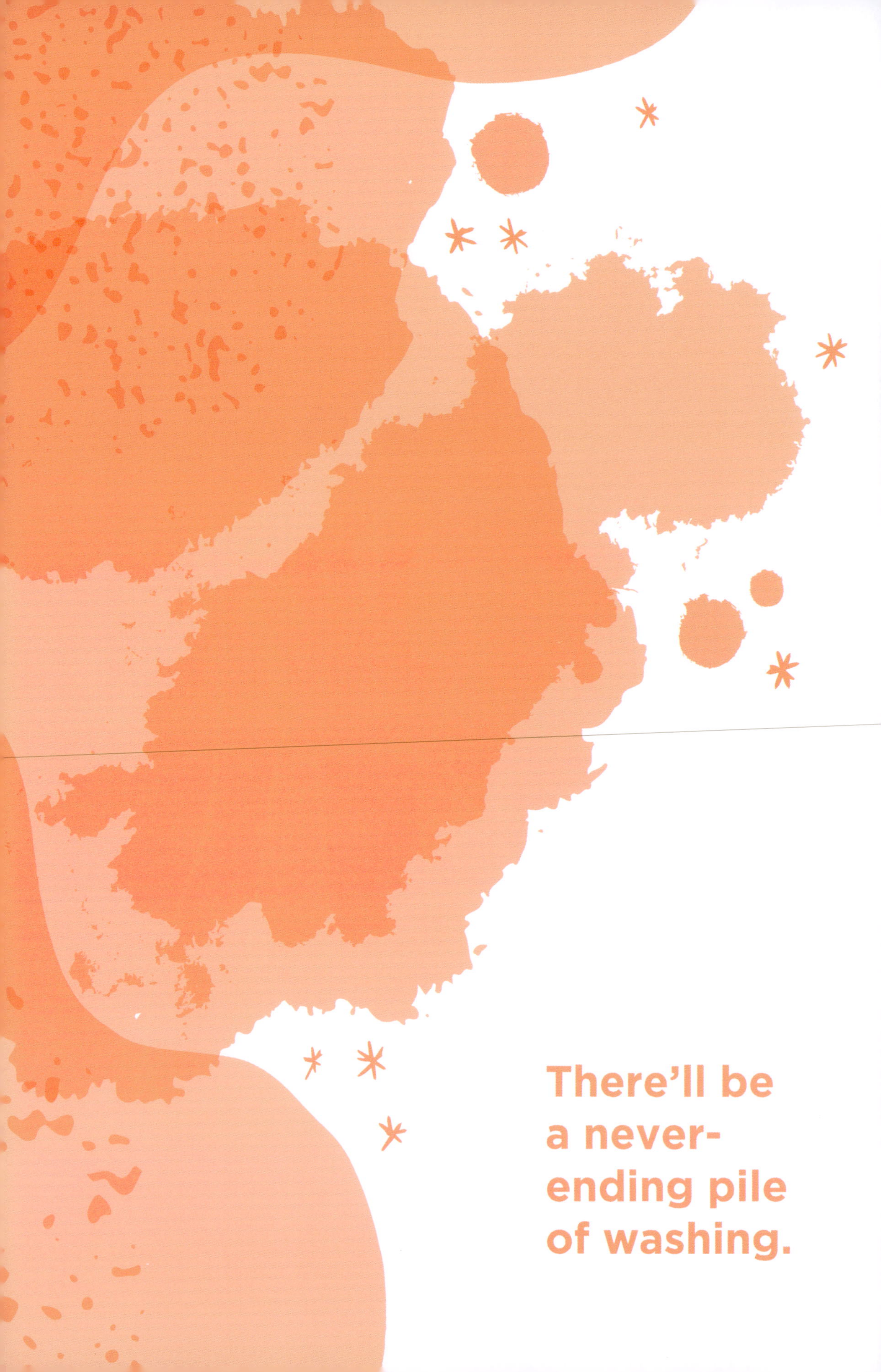

There'll be a never-ending pile of washing.

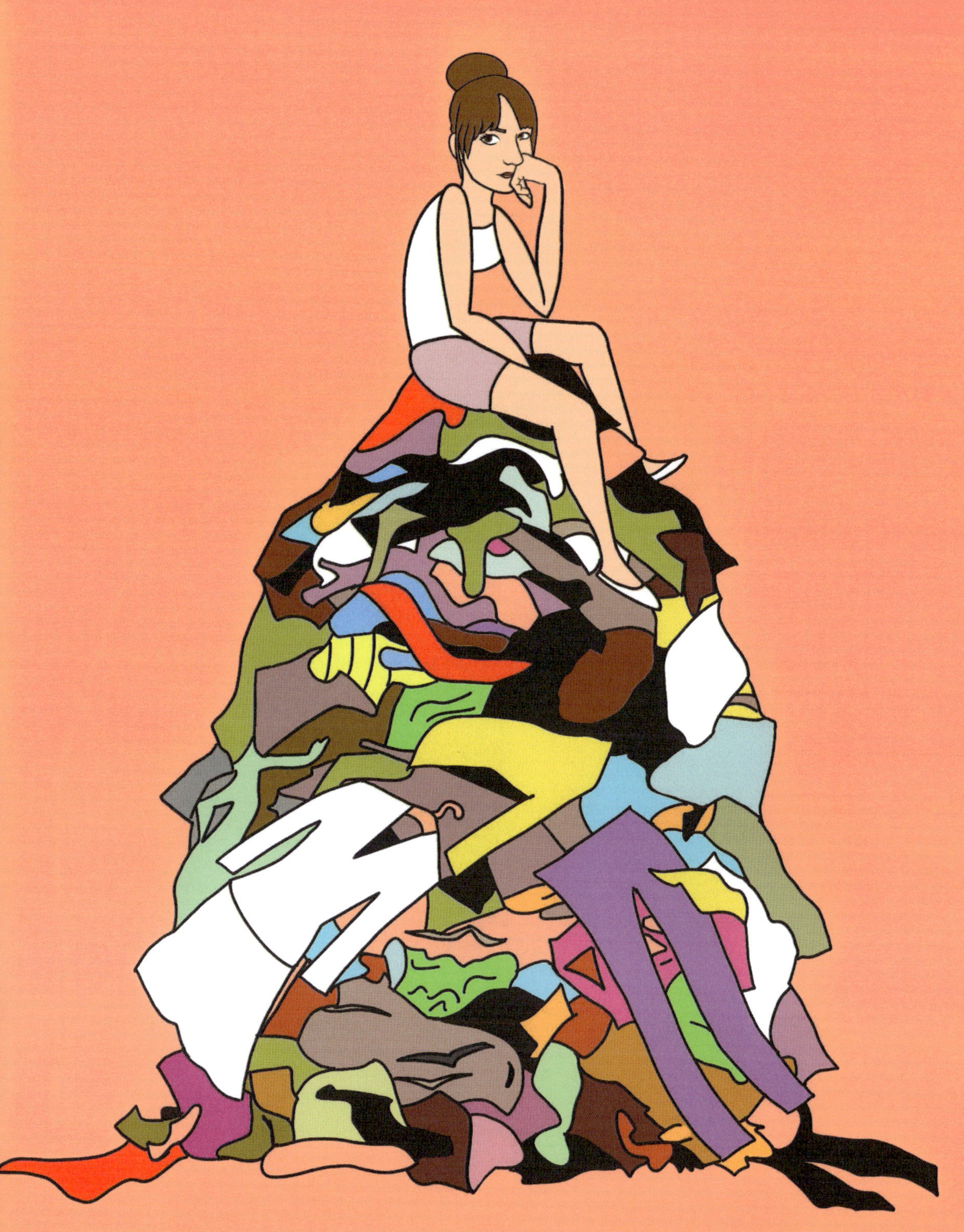

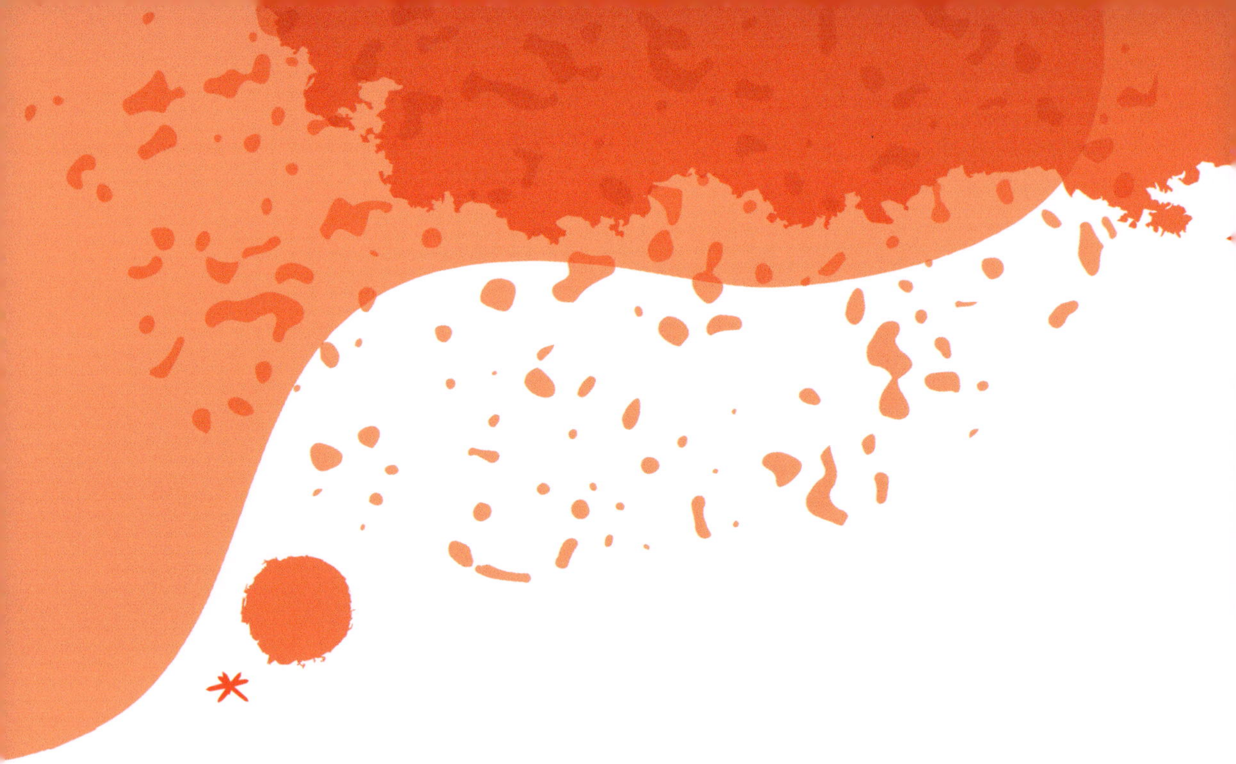

Your sleeves will turn red.

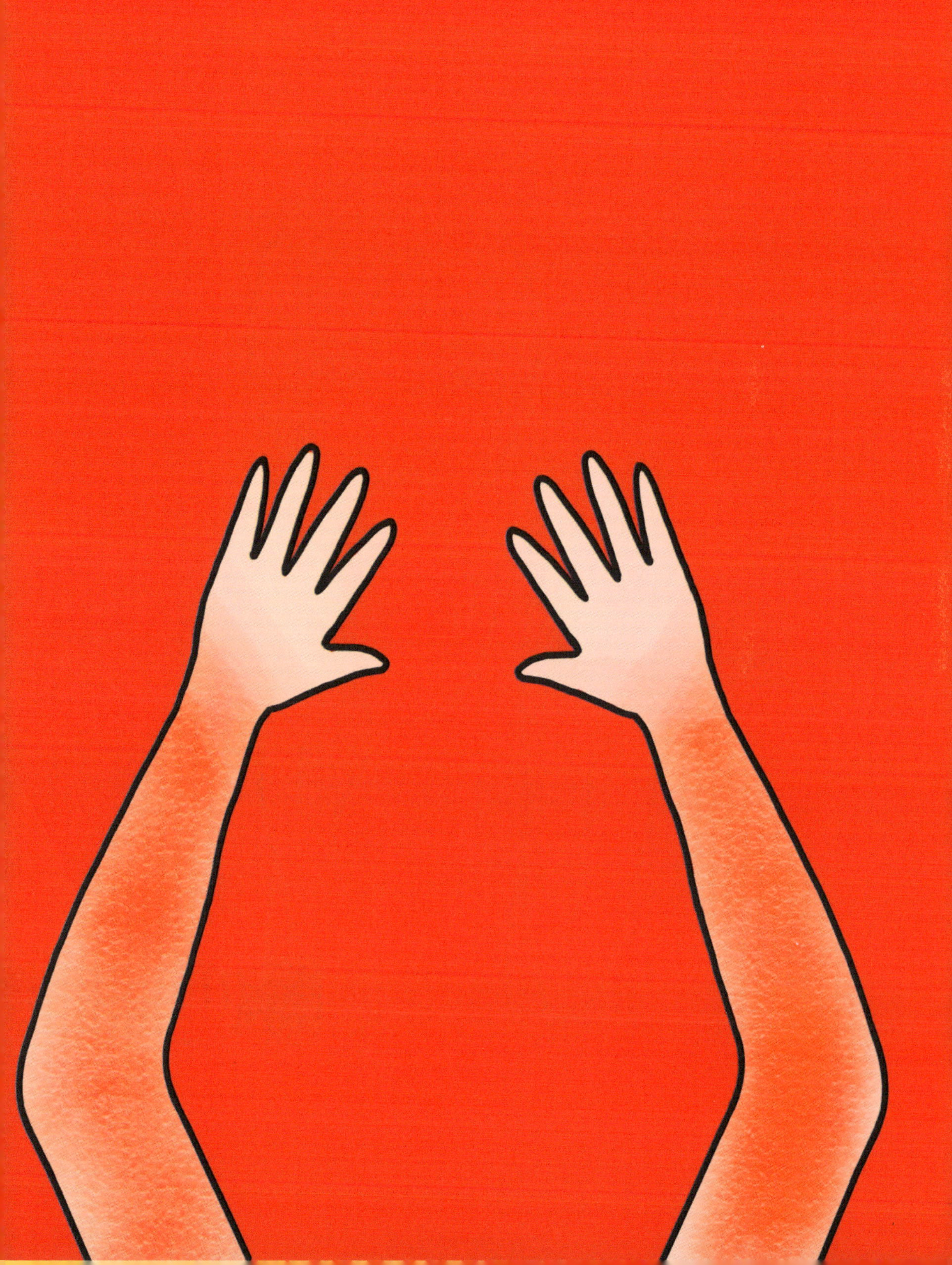

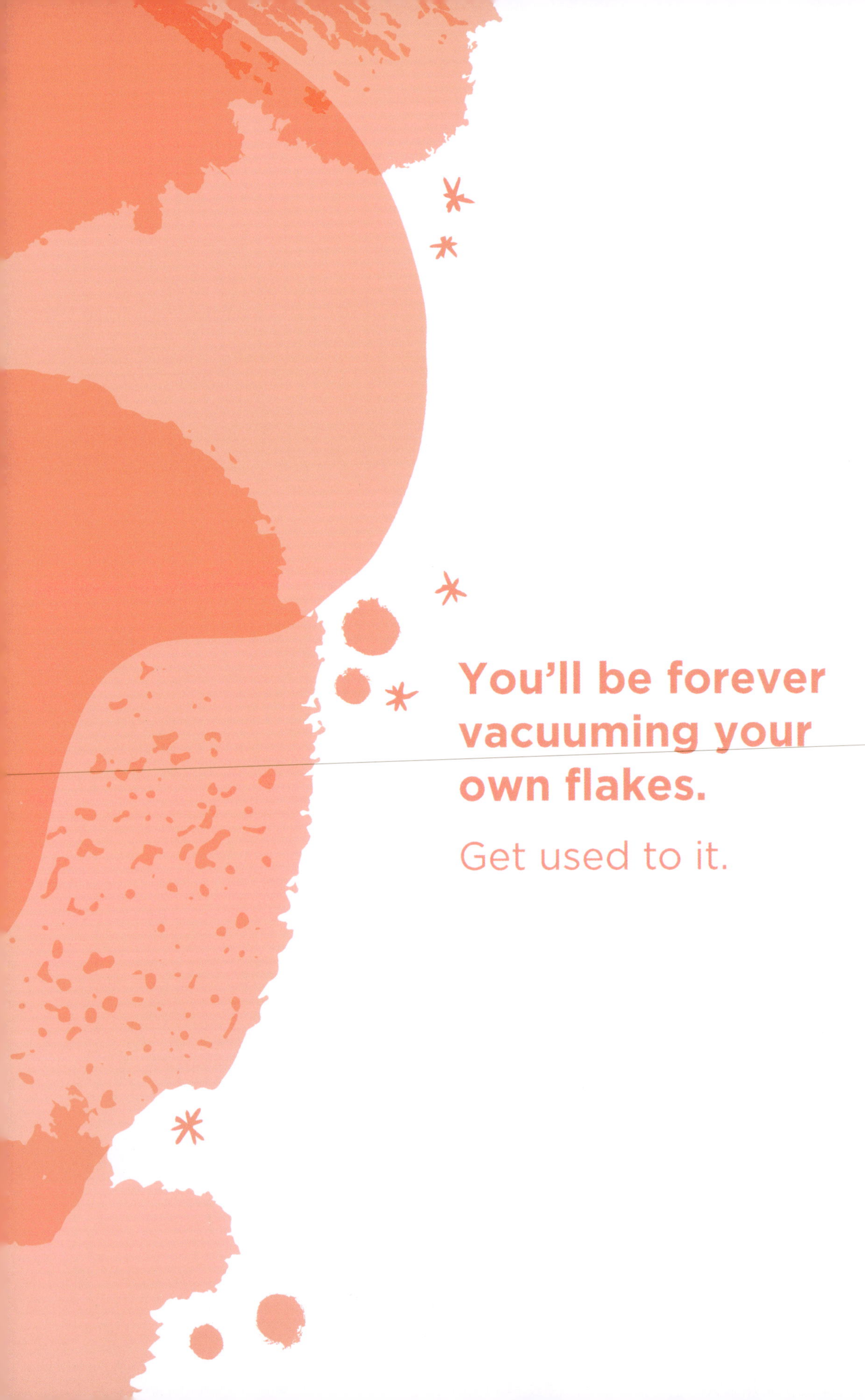

You'll be forever vacuuming your own flakes.

Get used to it.

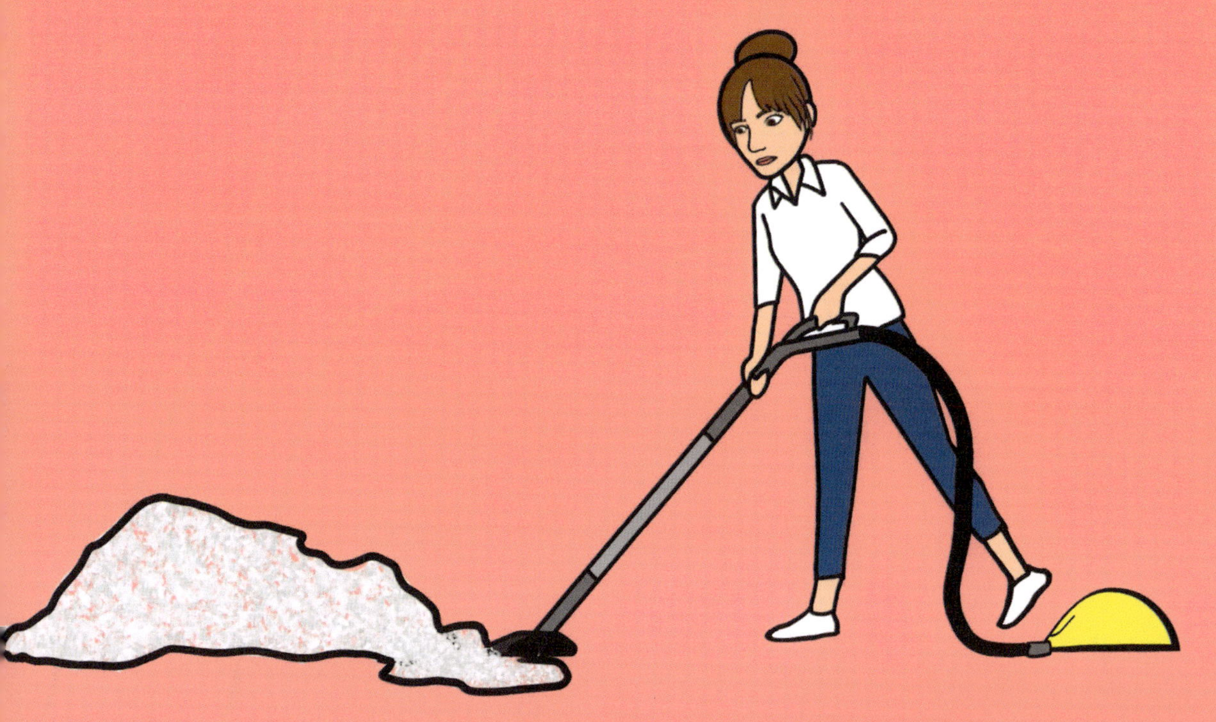

You'll do anything to avoid the dreaded sweat.

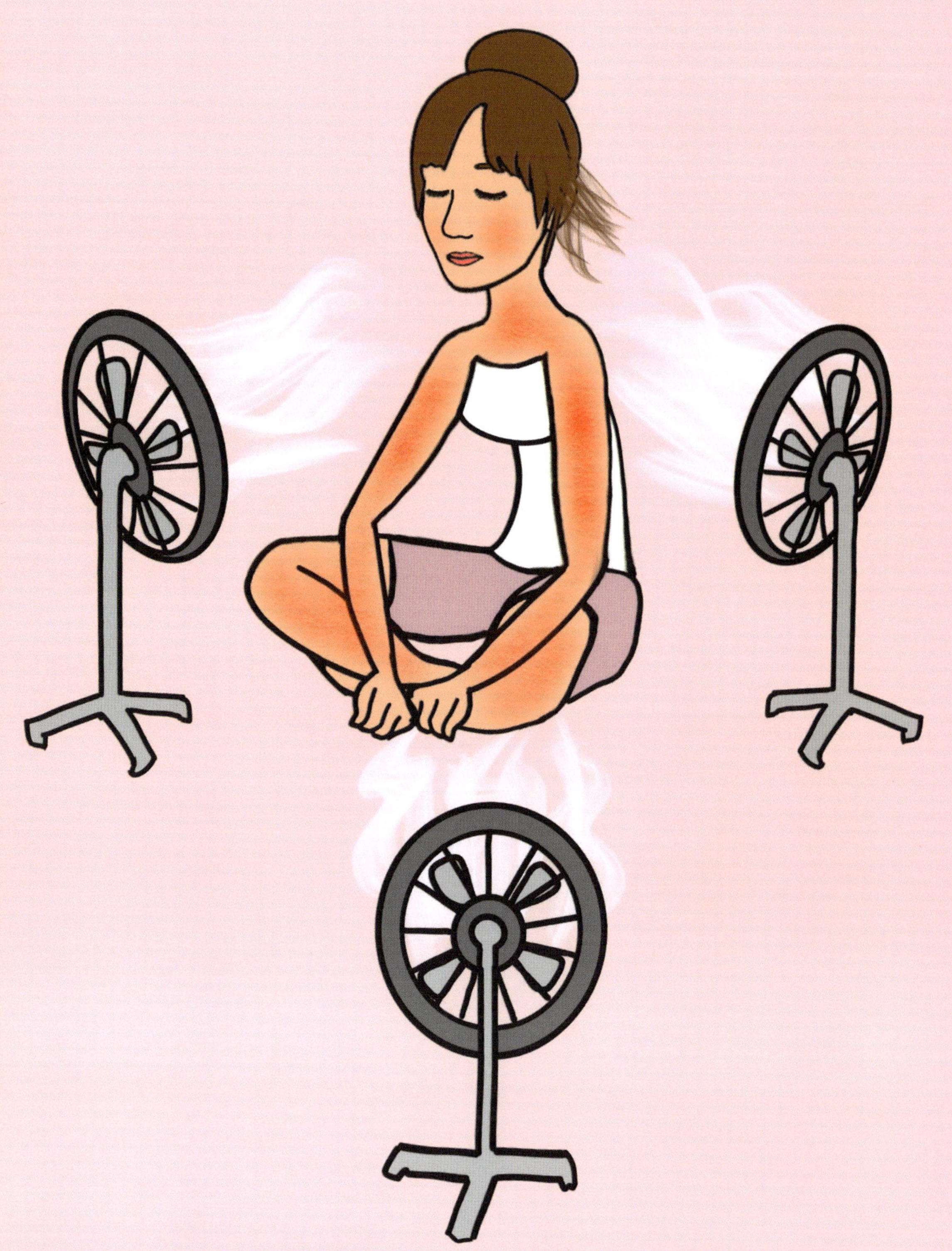

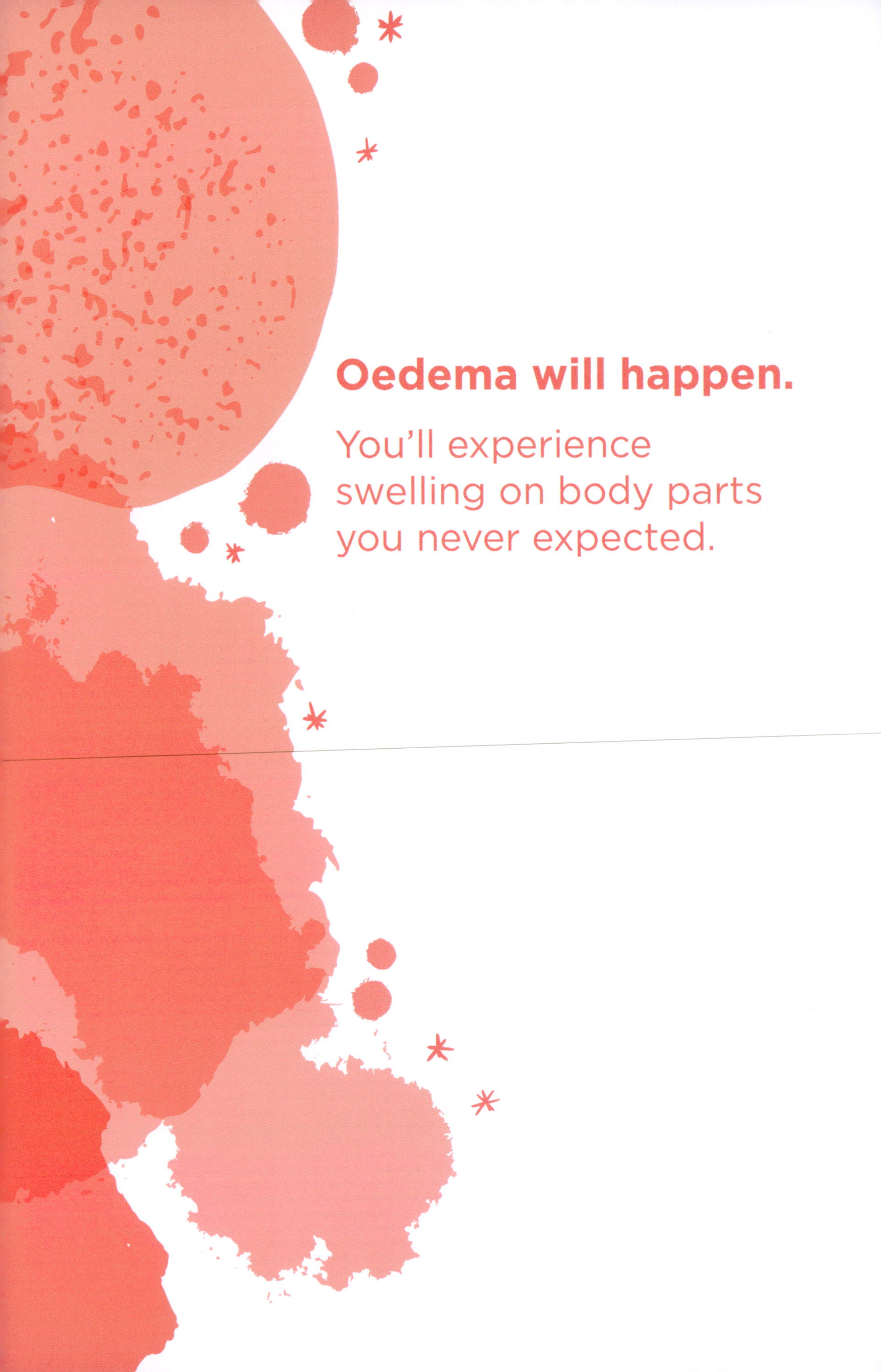

Oedema will happen.

You'll experience swelling on body parts you never expected.

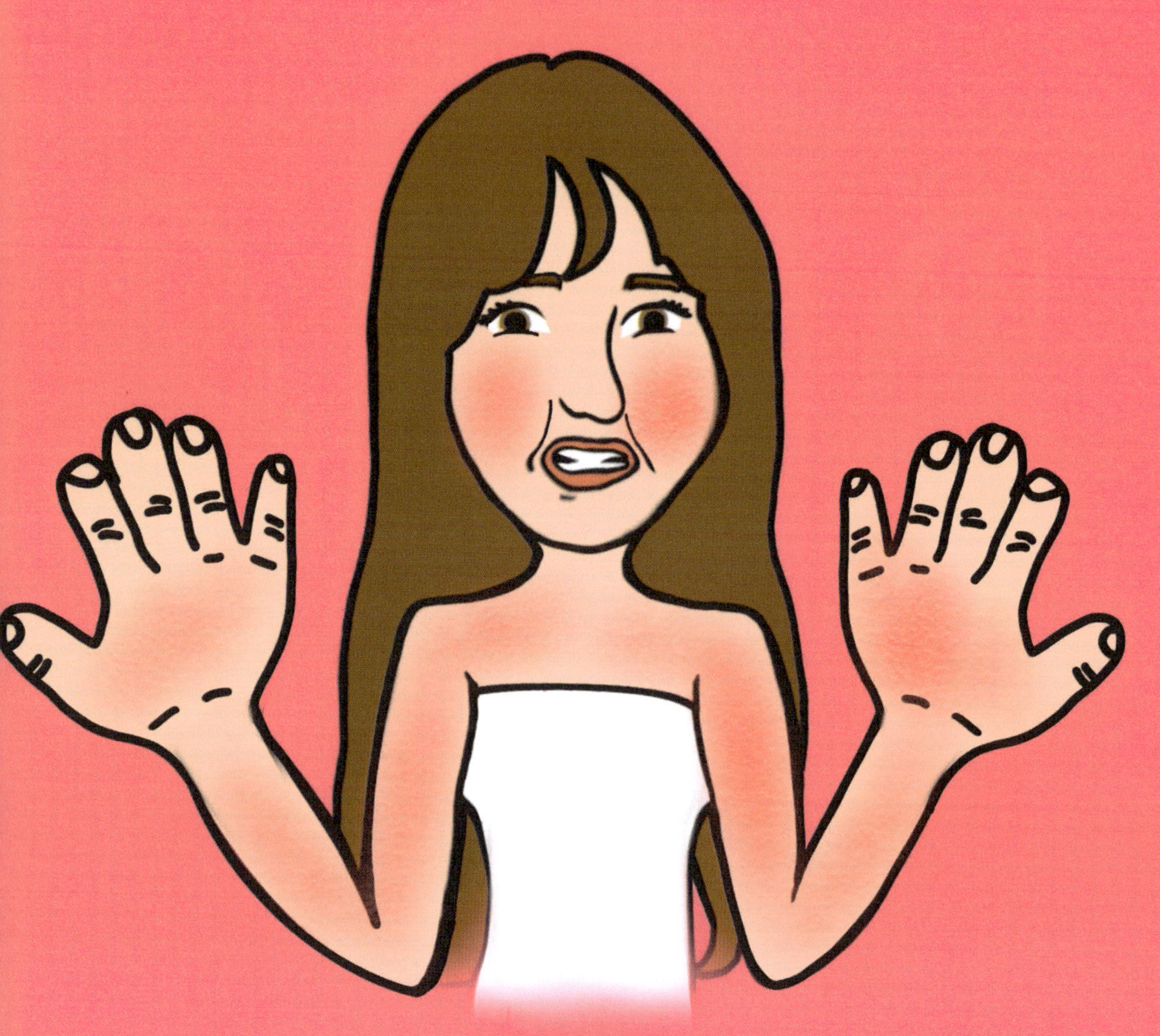

Skin hyperpigmentation is likely.

It can occur when using topical steroids and during recovery.

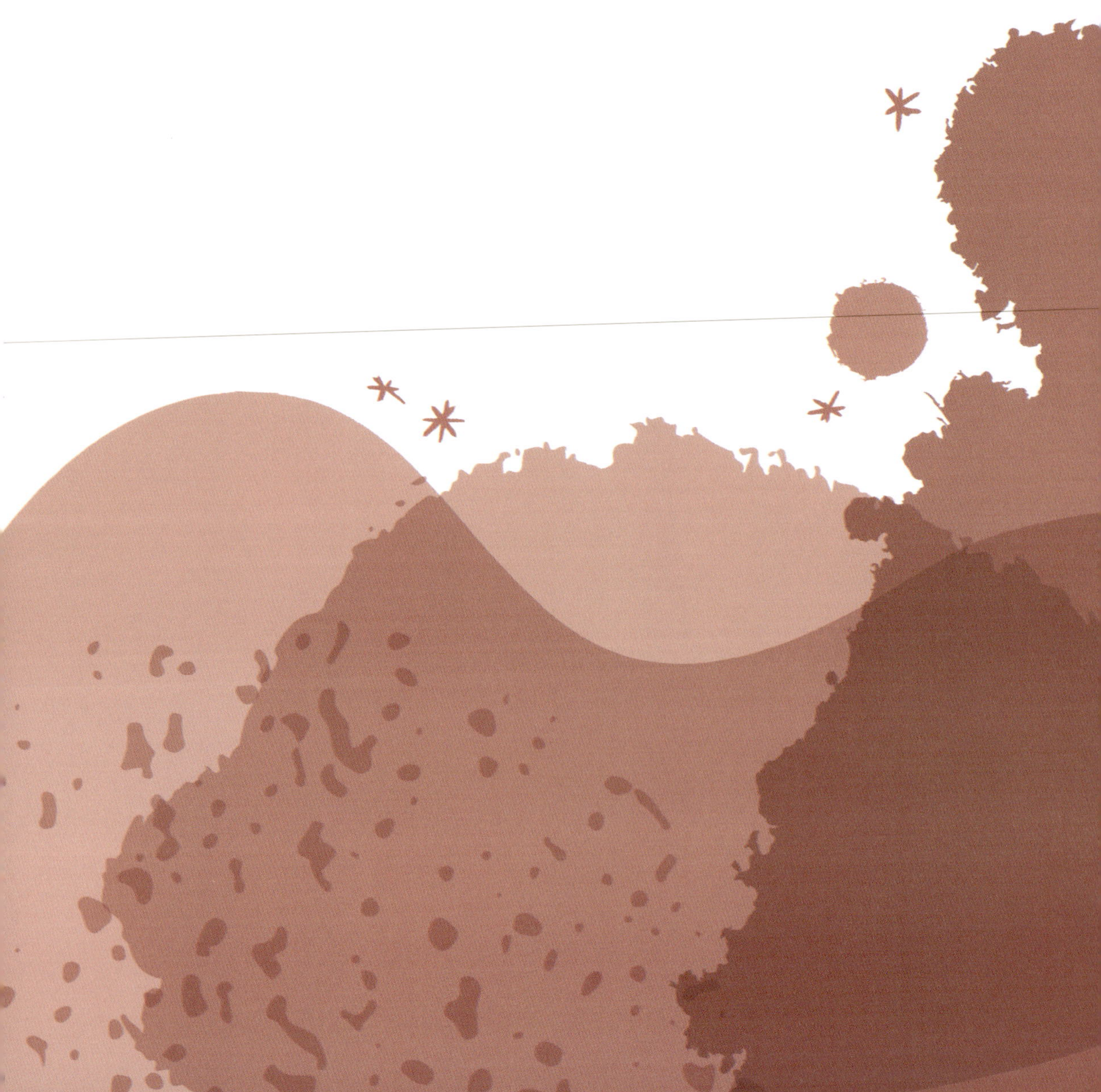

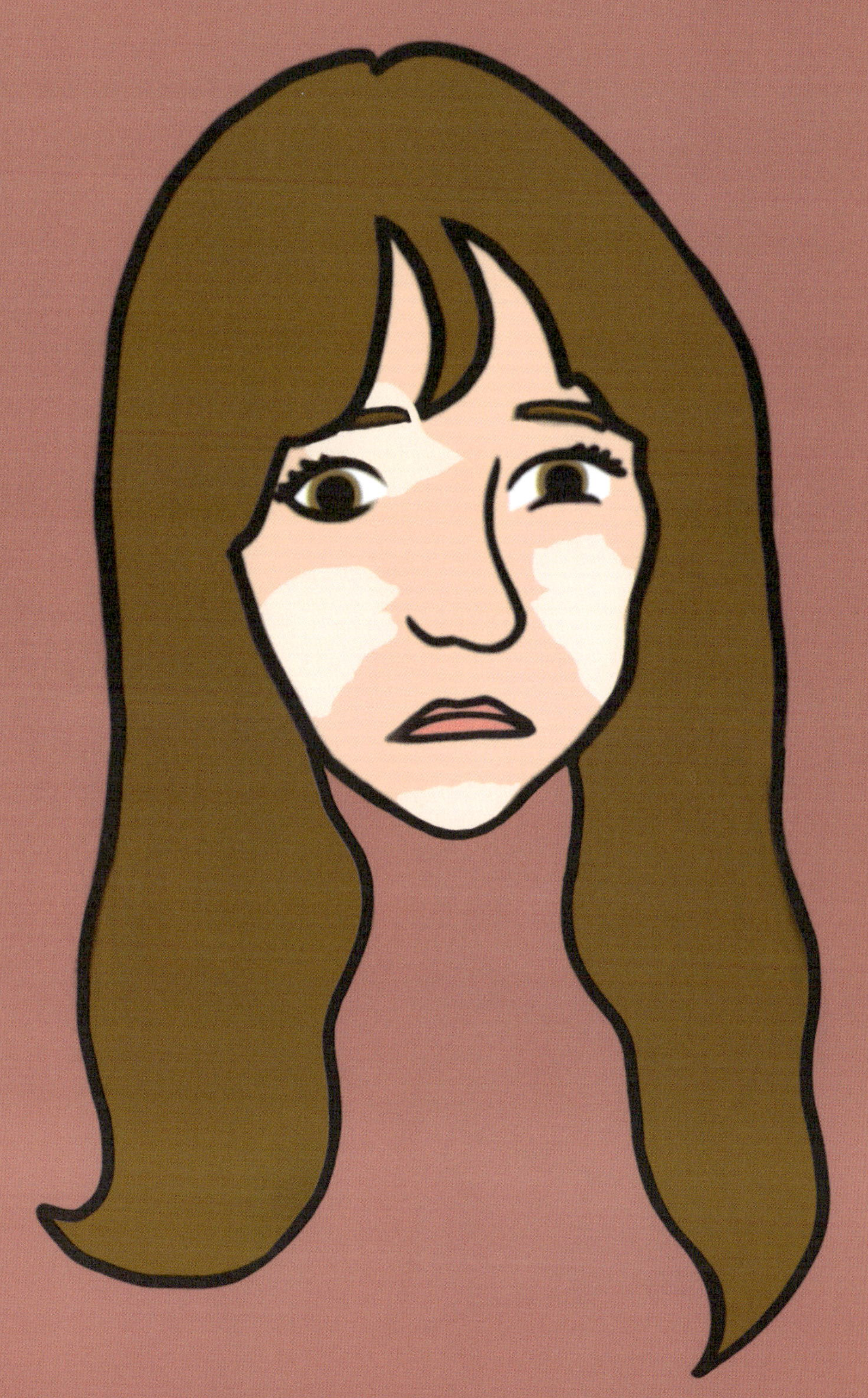

You’ll experience hair loss.

In new places.

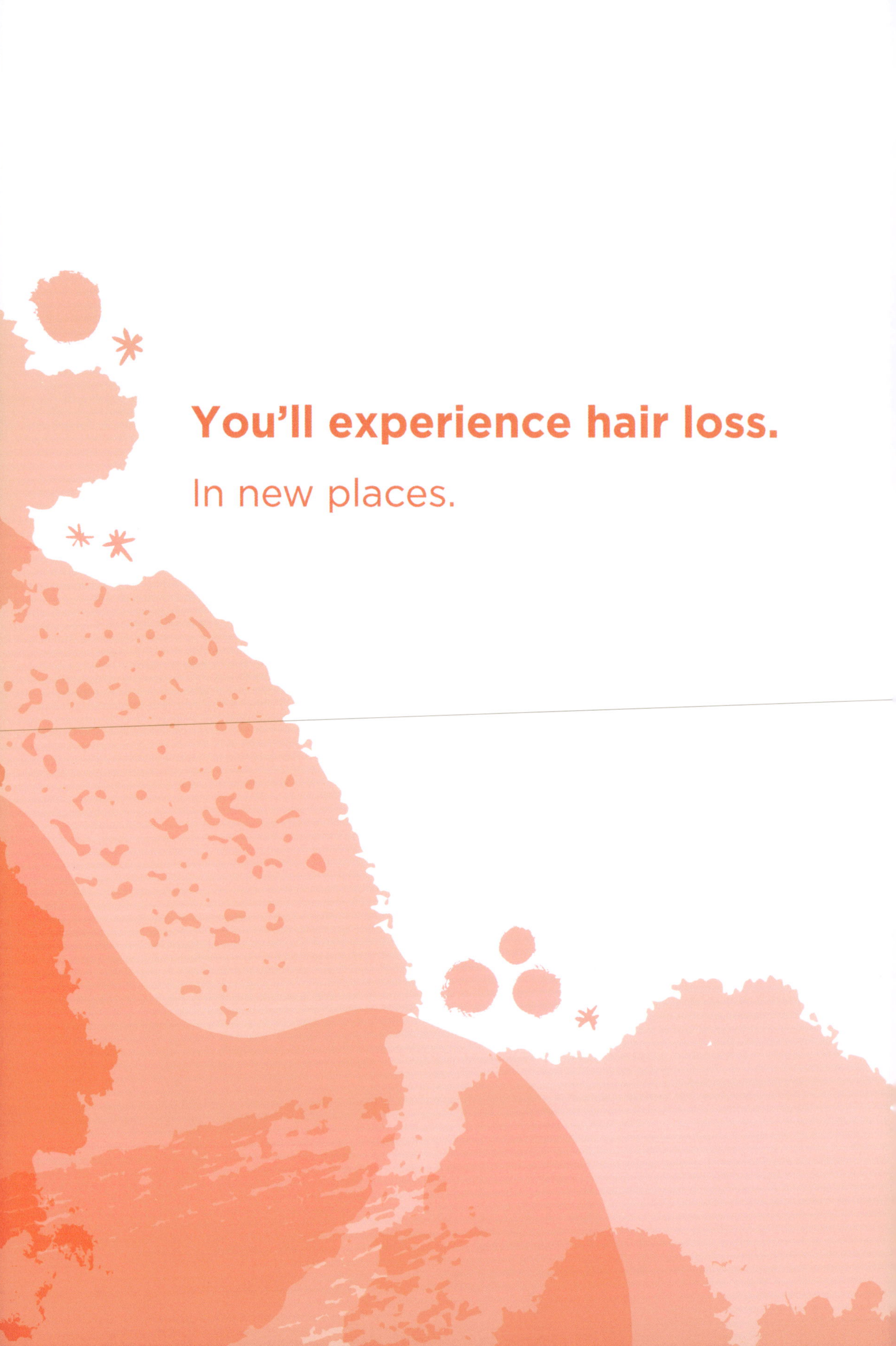

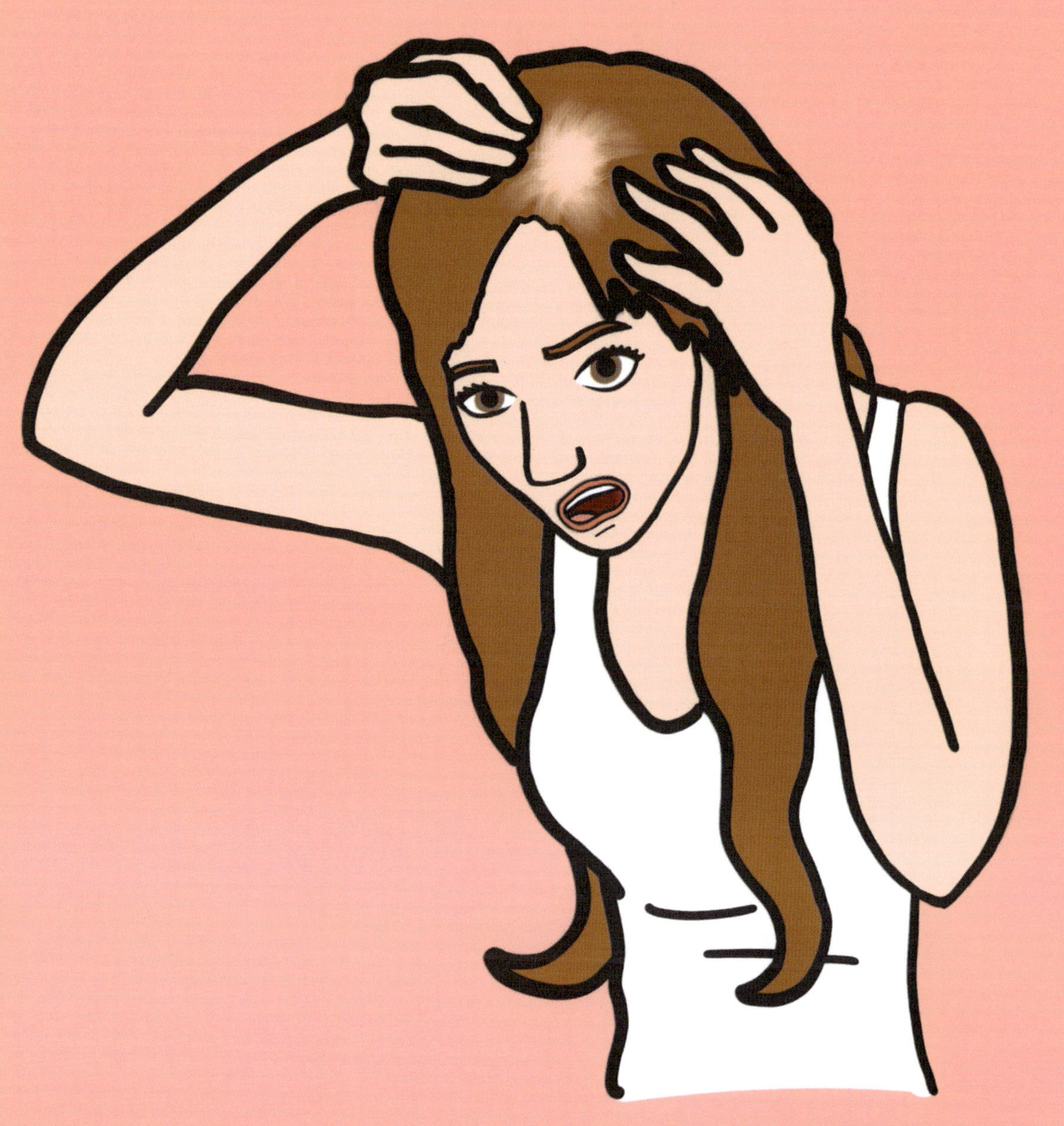

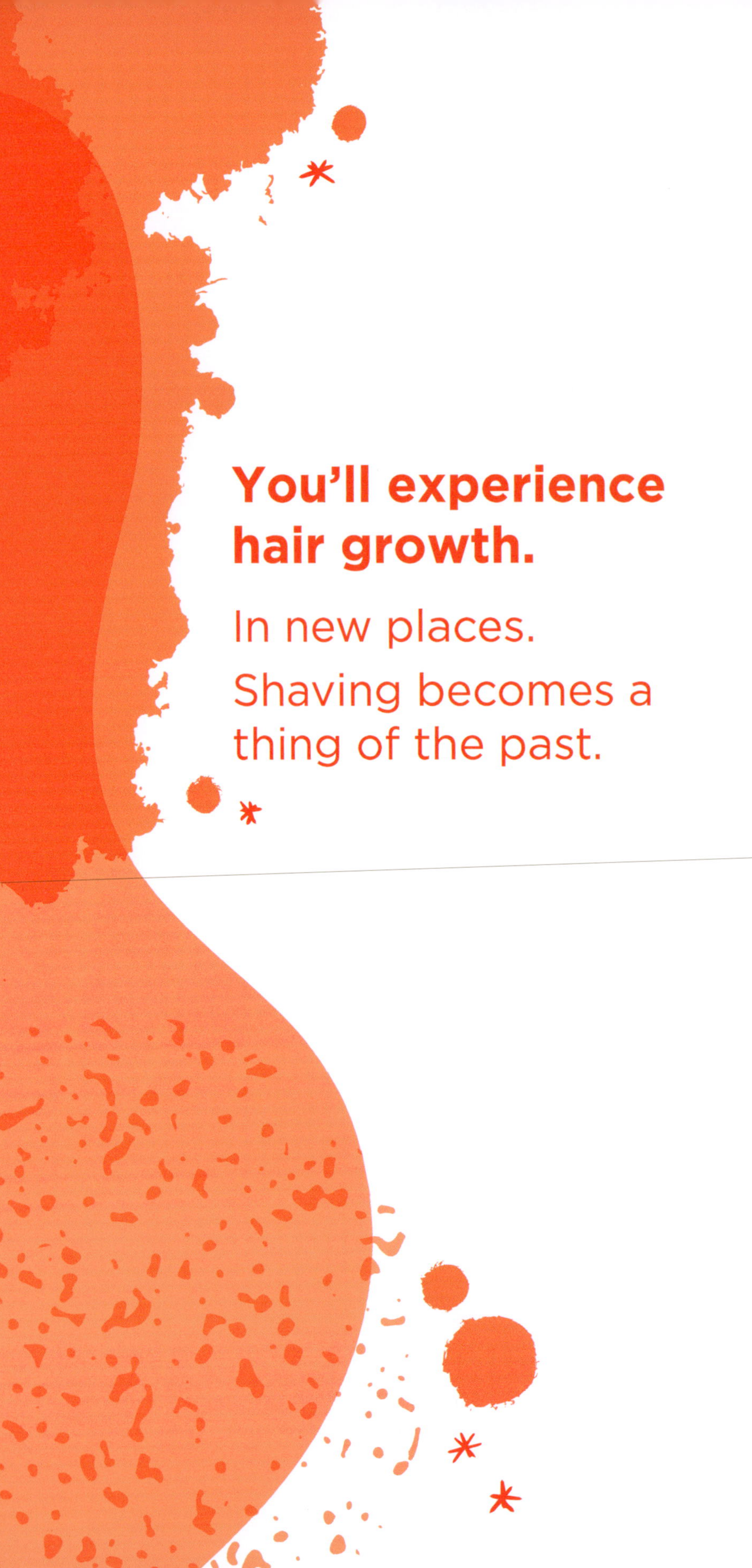

You'll experience hair growth.

In new places.

Shaving becomes a thing of the past.

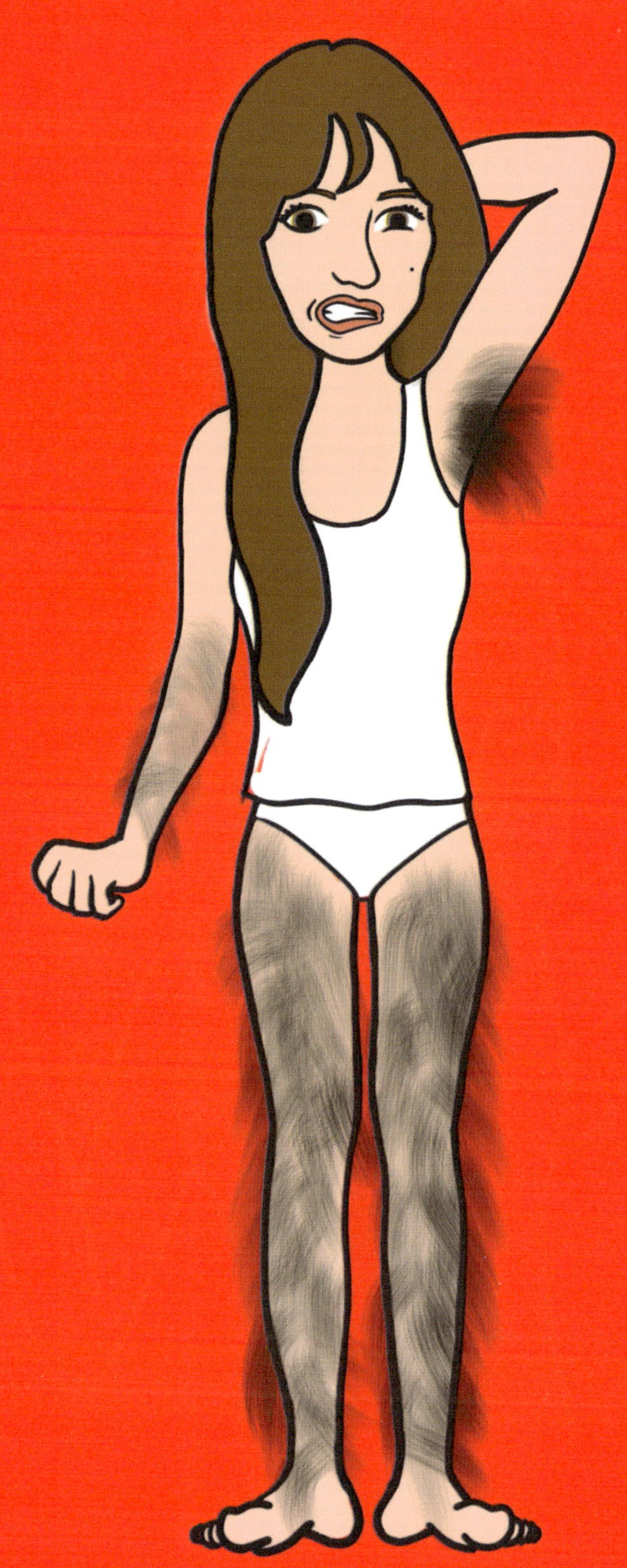

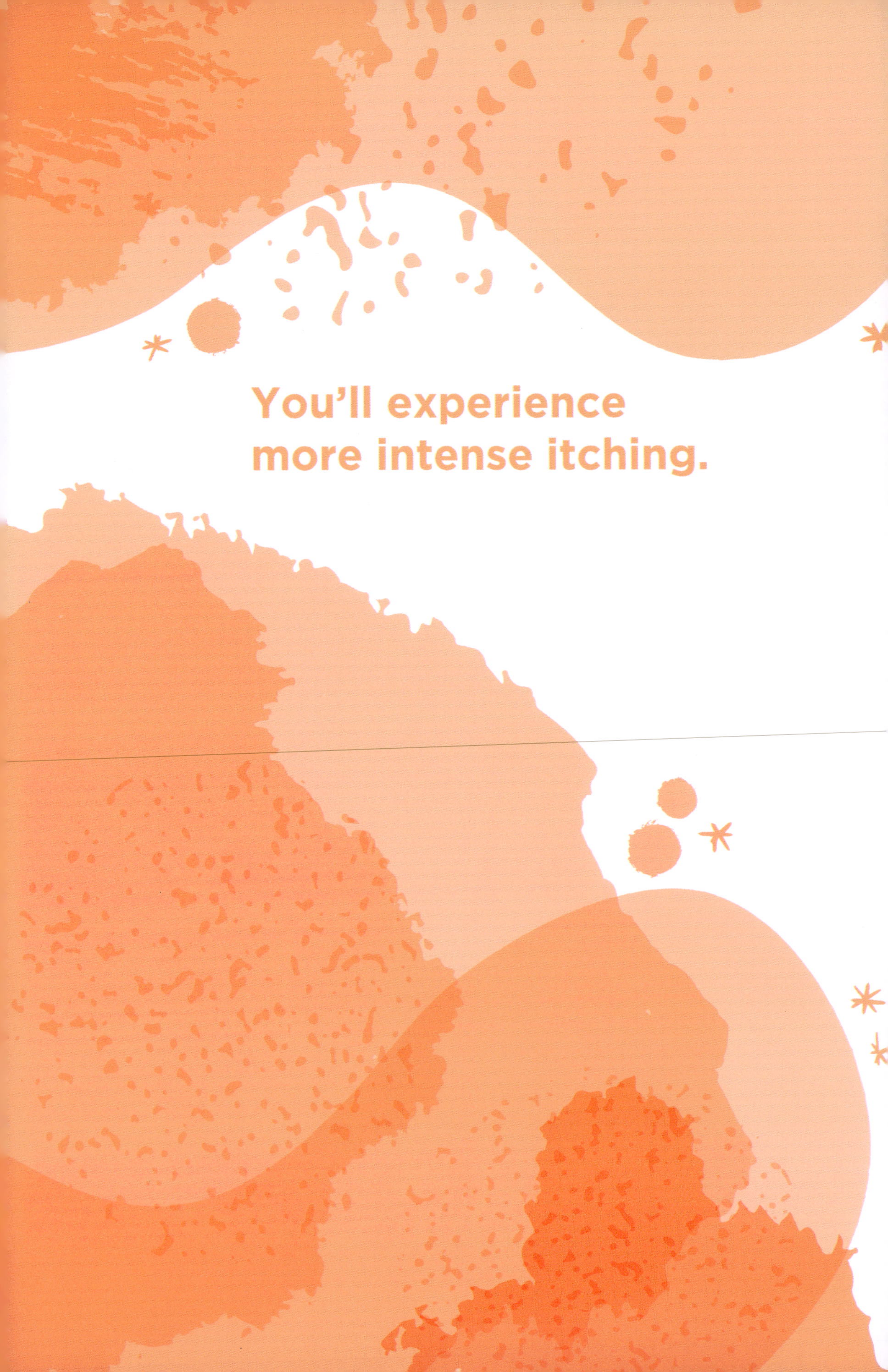
You'll experience
more intense itching.

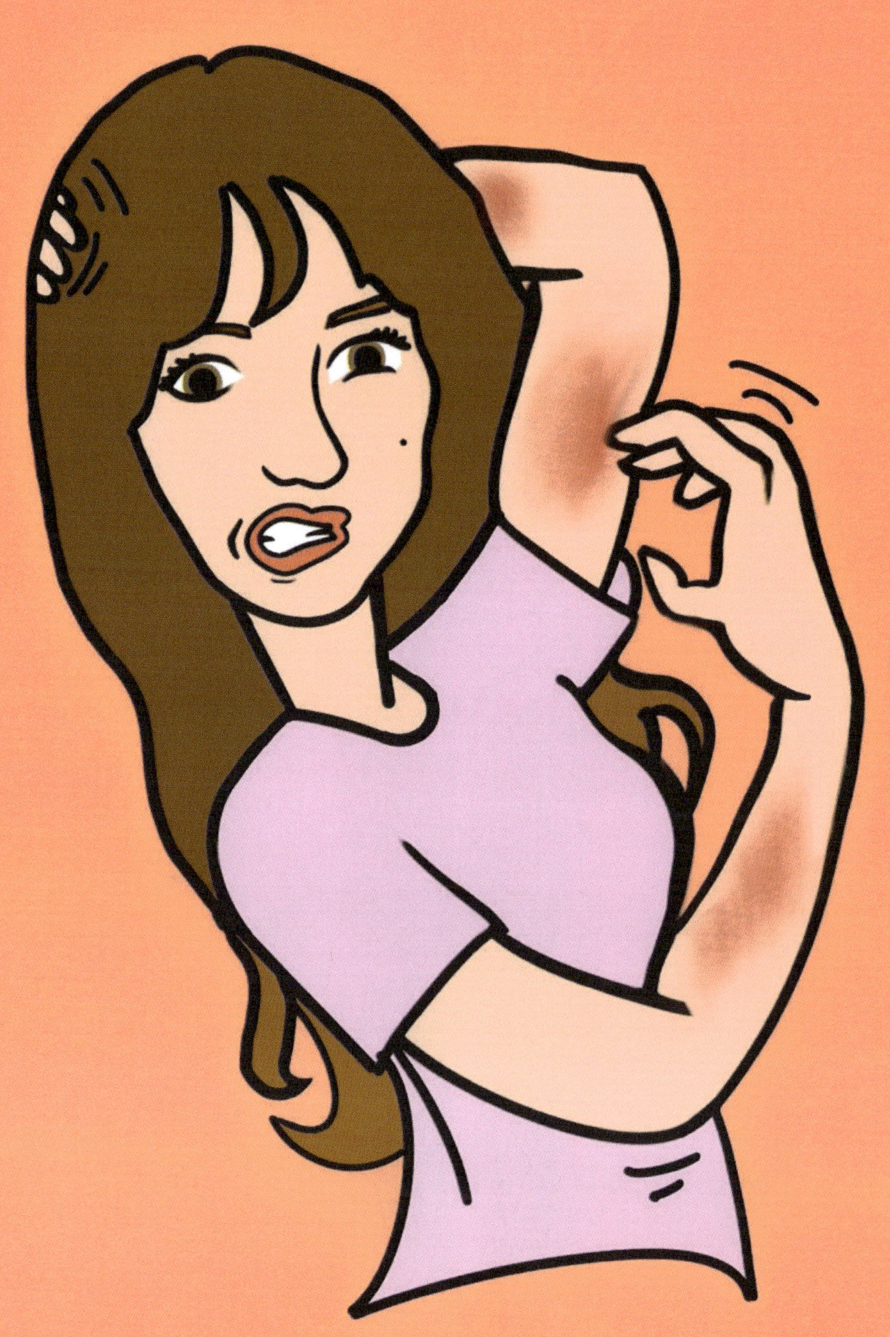

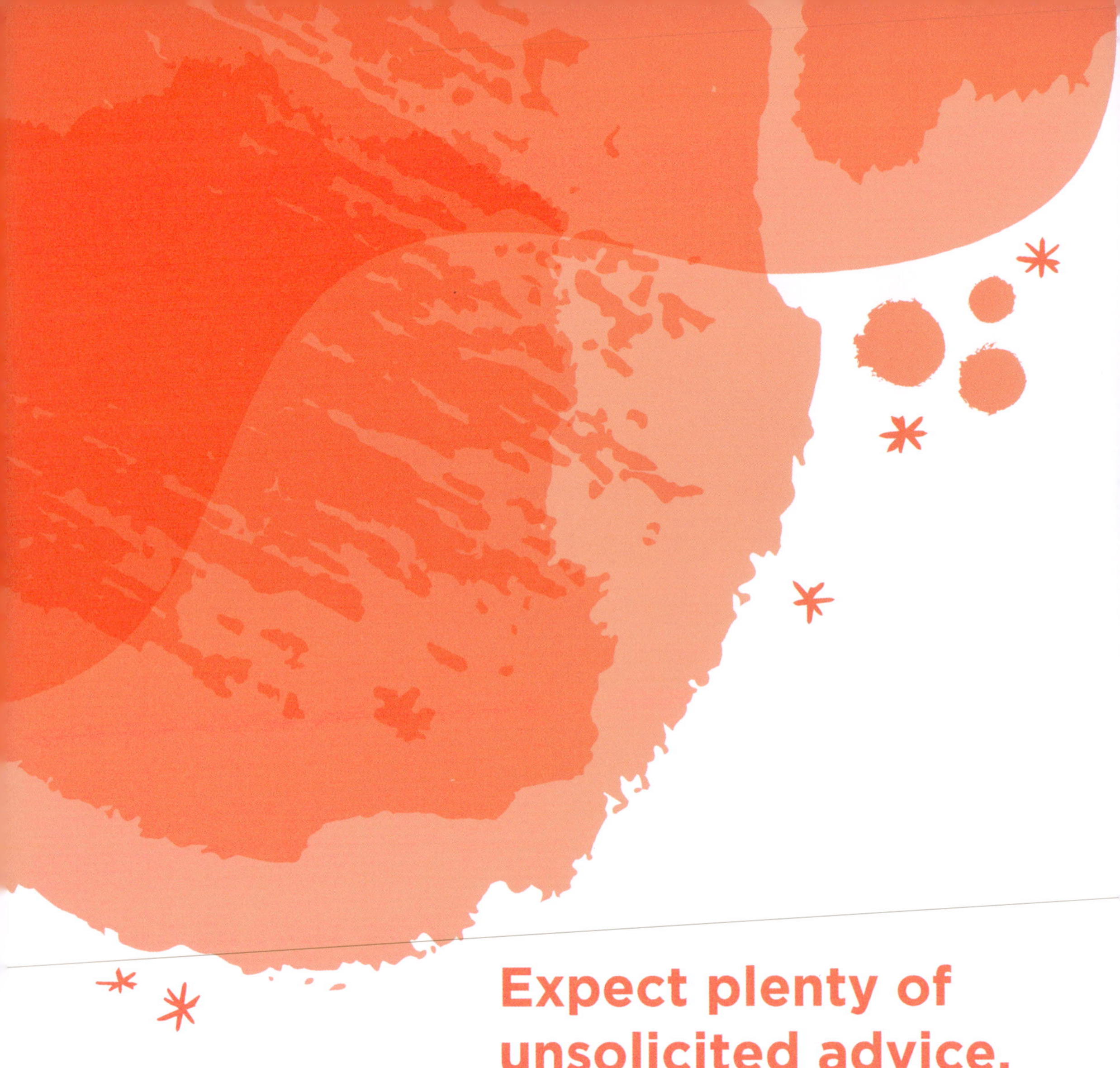

Expect plenty of unsolicited advice.

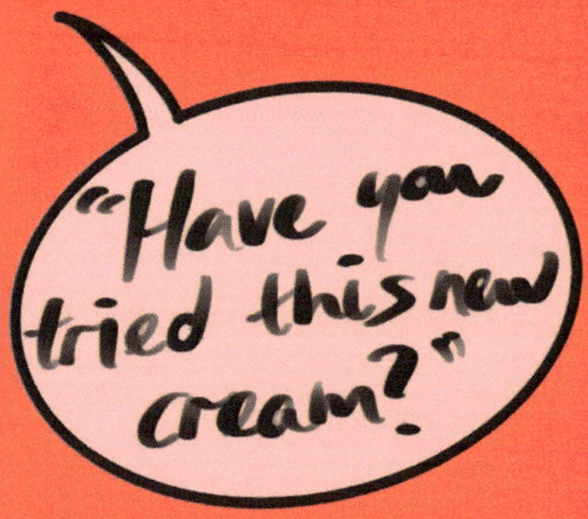
"Have you tried this new cream?"

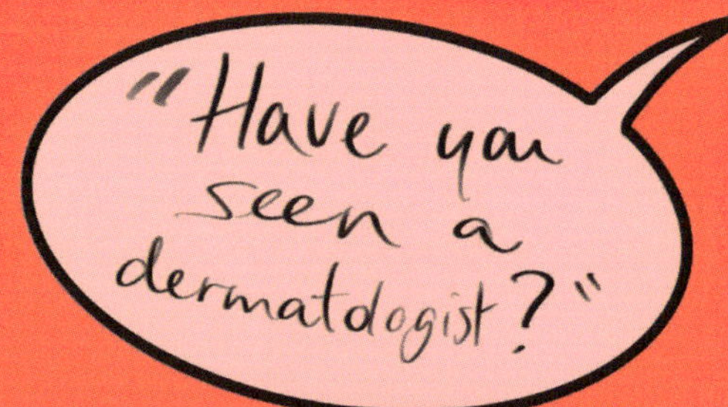
"Have you seen a dermatdogist?"

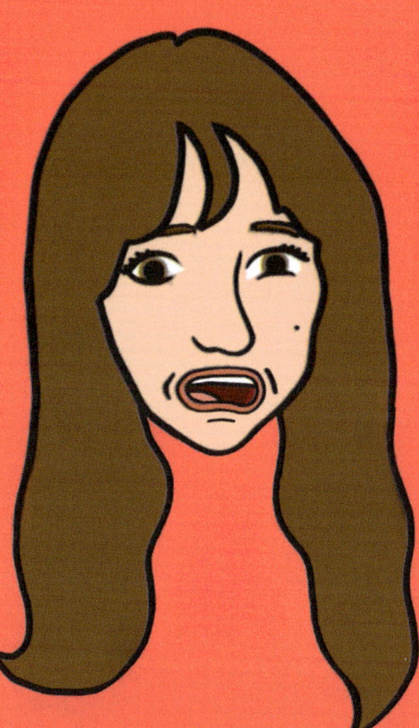
"Why don't you give up wheat?"
"Try drinking celery Juice!"
"Have you used camel milk?"
"Have you tried just not scratching?

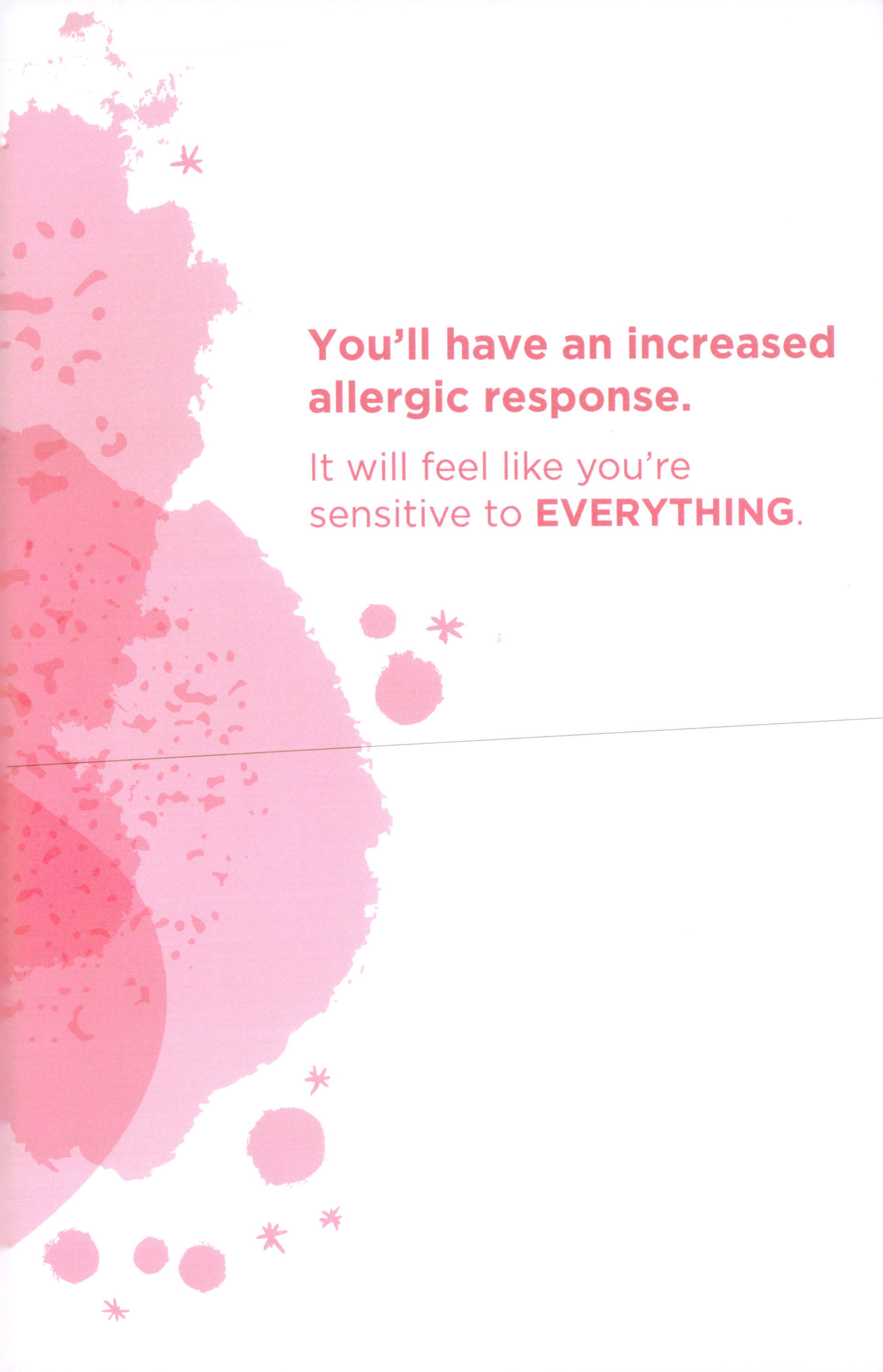

You'll have an increased allergic response.

It will feel like you're sensitive to **EVERYTHING**.

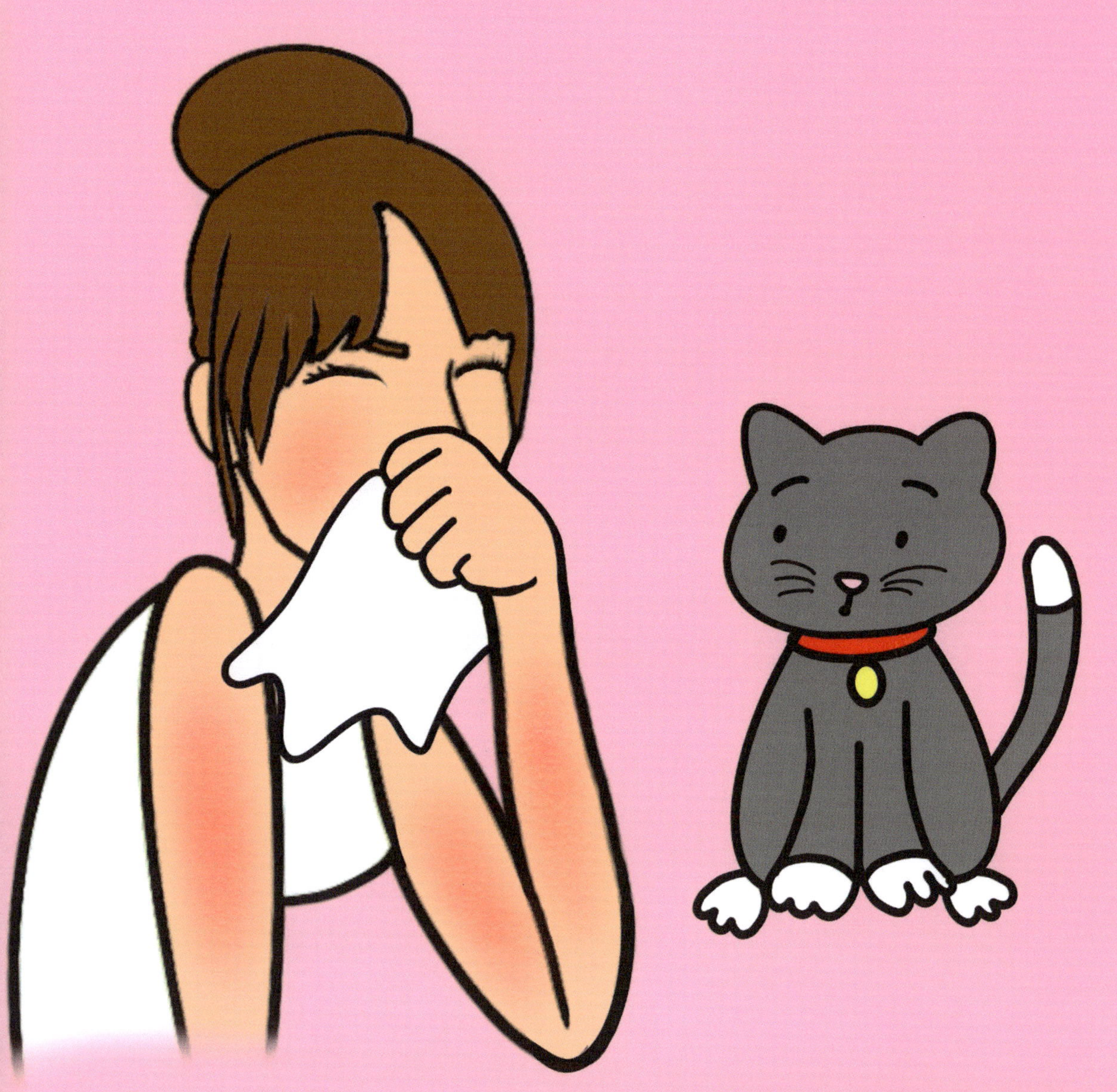

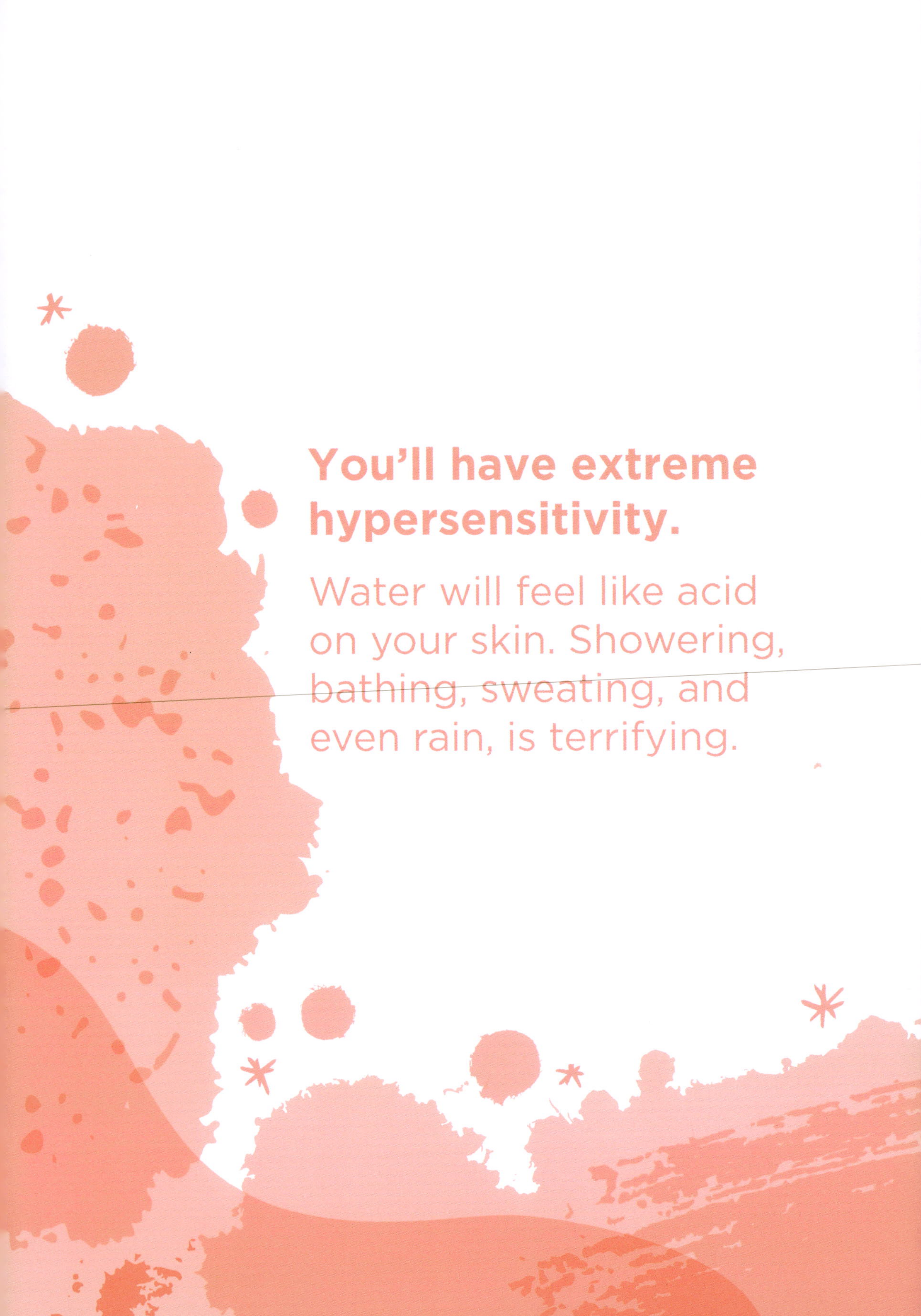

You'll have extreme hypersensitivity.

Water will feel like acid on your skin. Showering, bathing, sweating, and even rain, is terrifying.

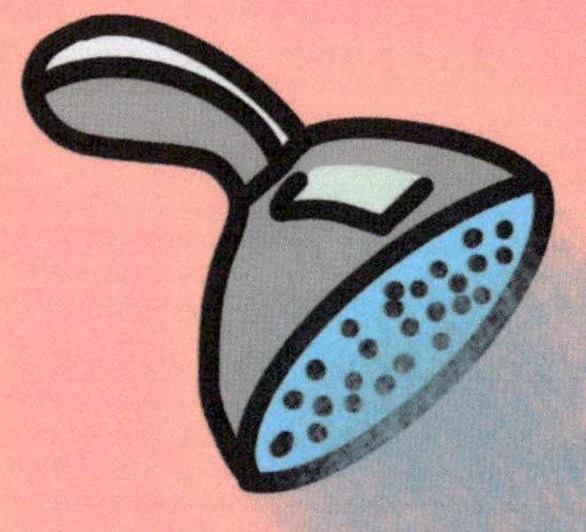

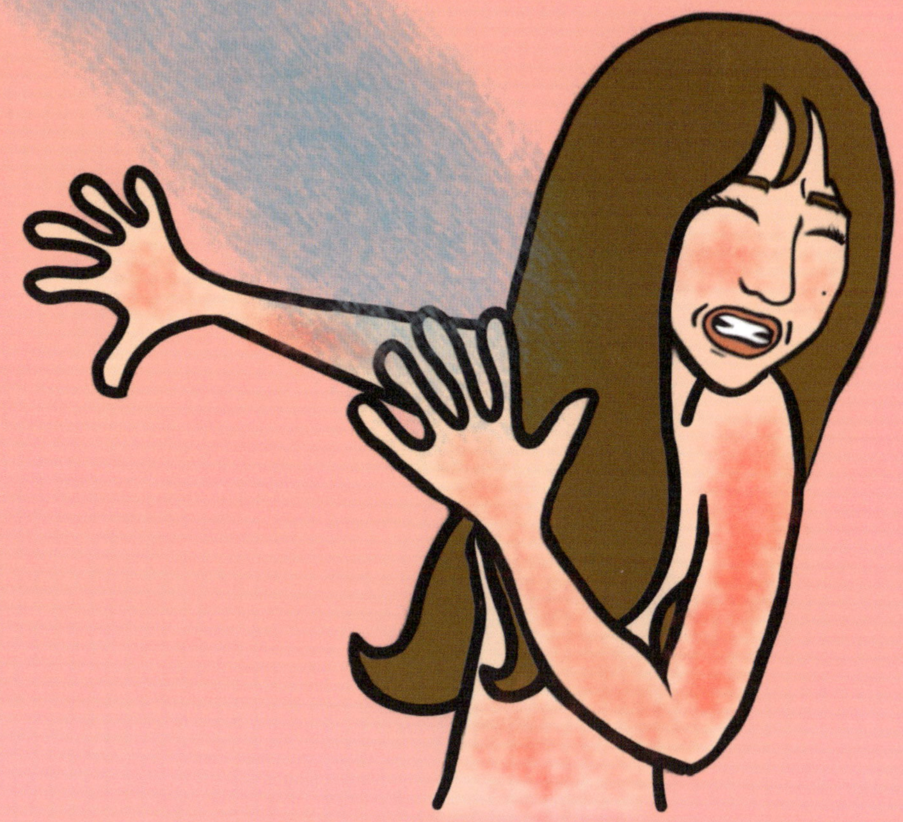

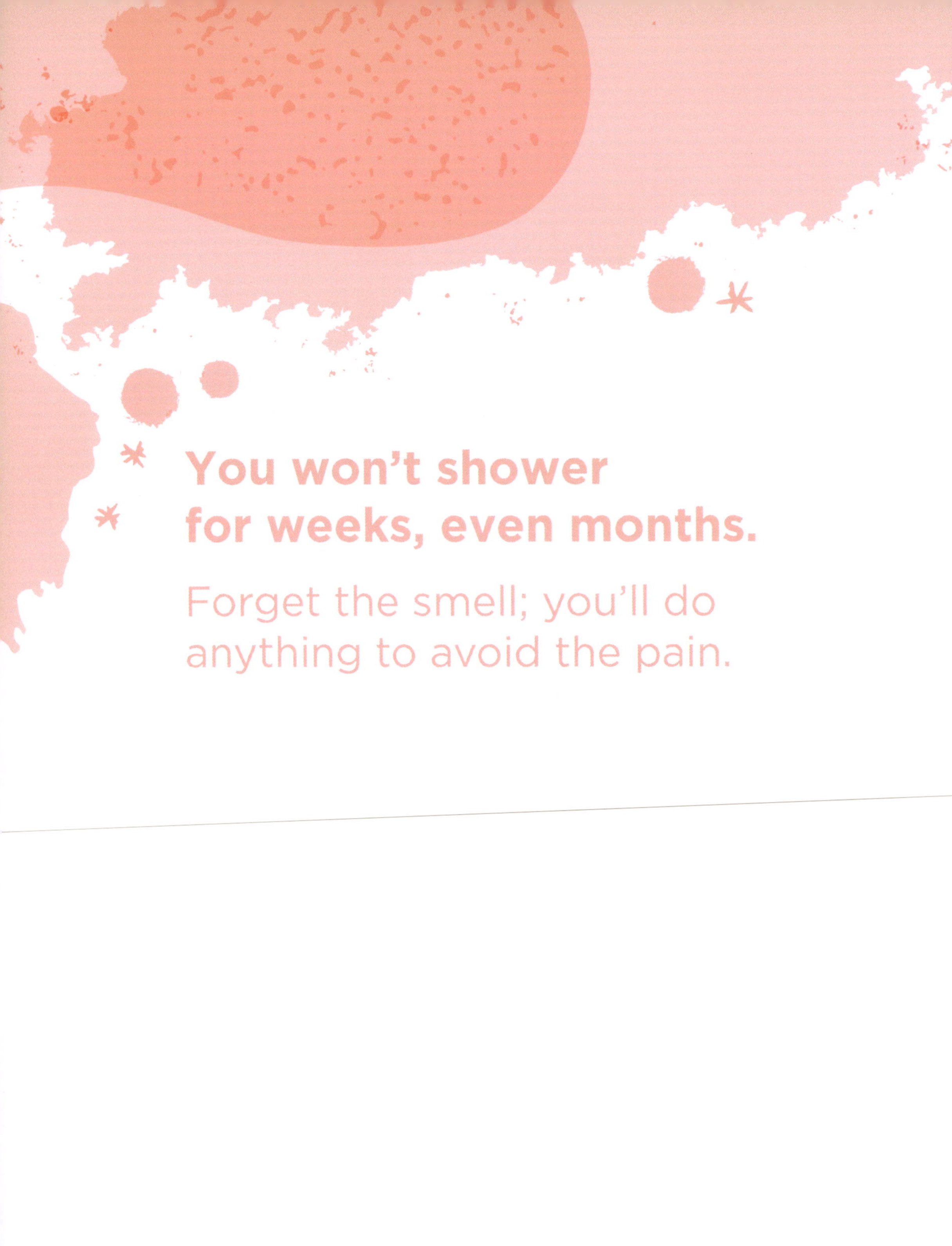

You won’t shower for weeks, even months.

Forget the smell; you’ll do anything to avoid the pain.

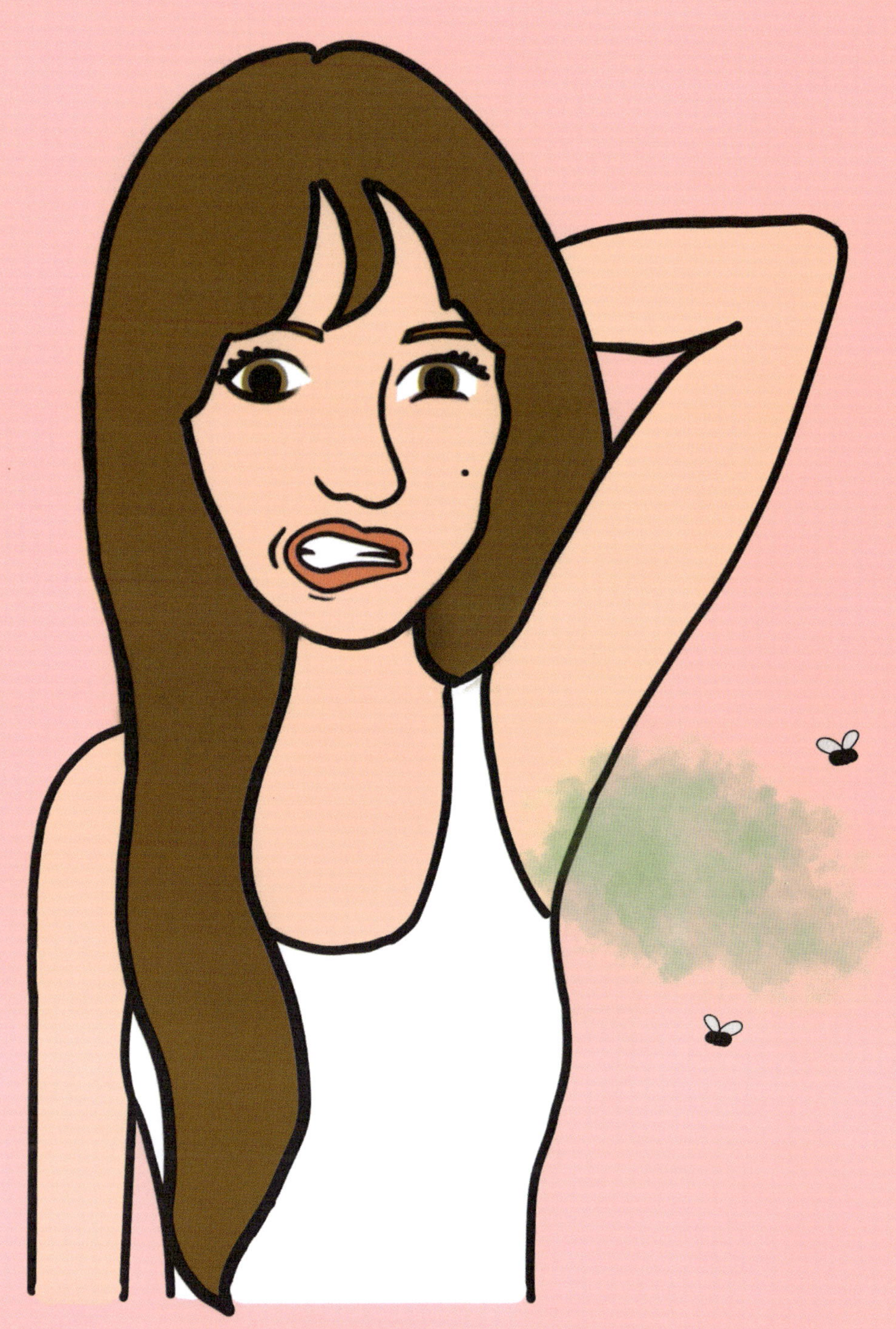

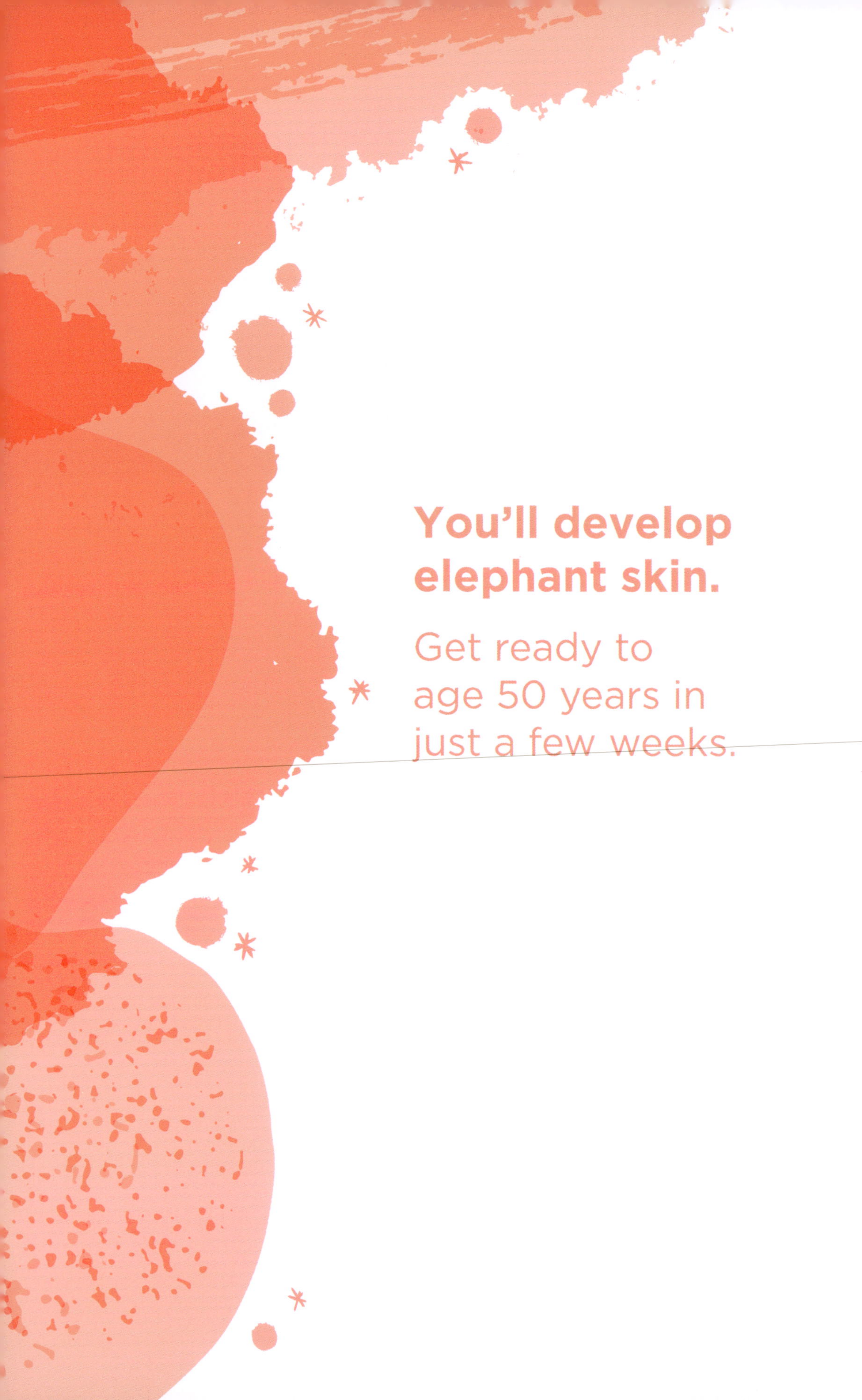

You'll develop elephant skin.

Get ready to age 50 years in just a few weeks.

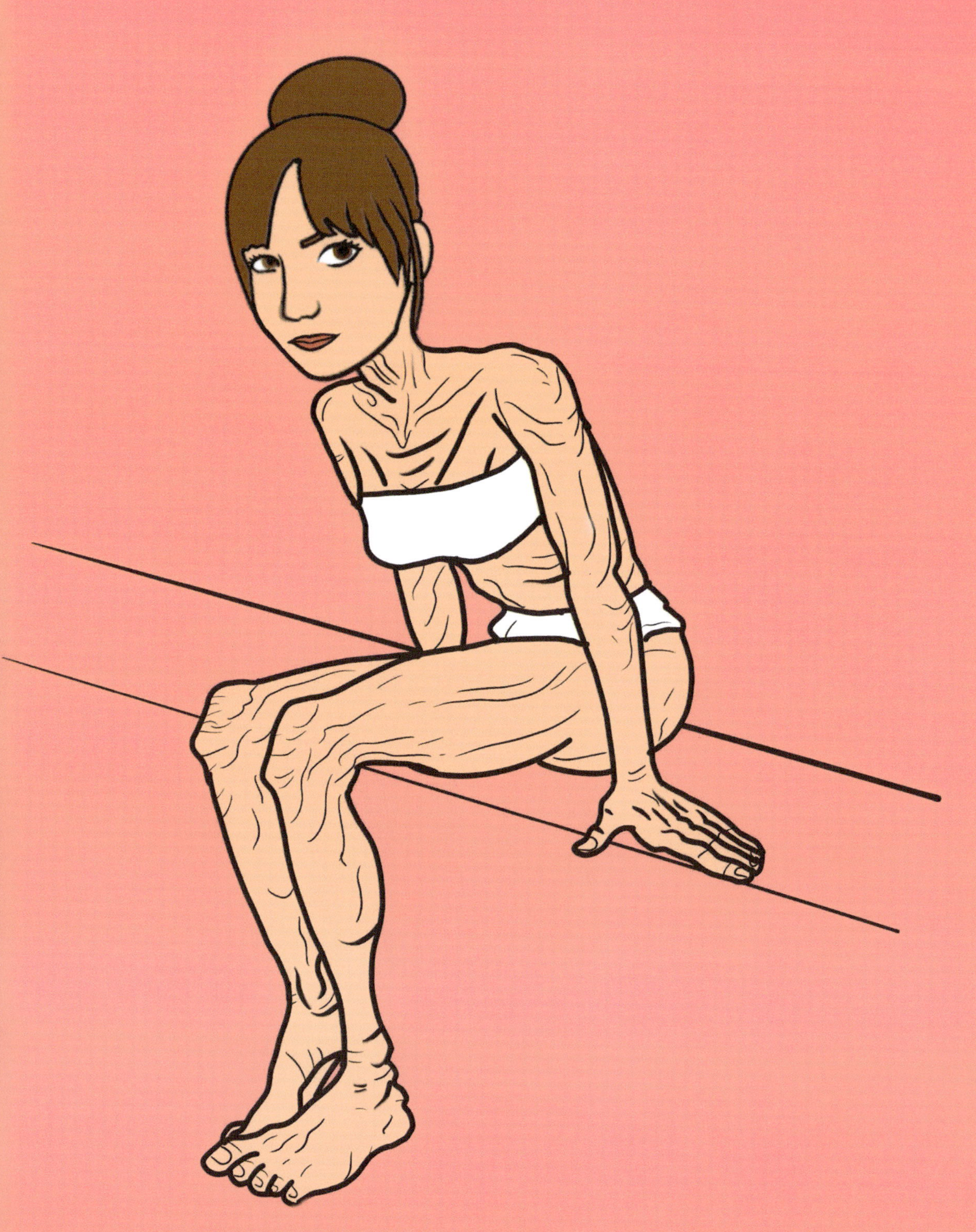

It will feel like waking up in a sandpit every day.

There'll be enough skin flakes to make a beach.

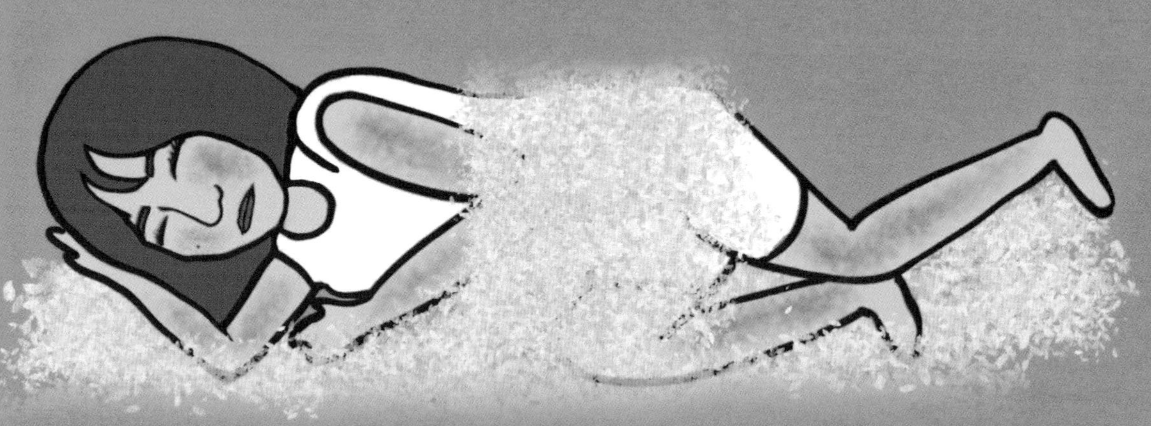

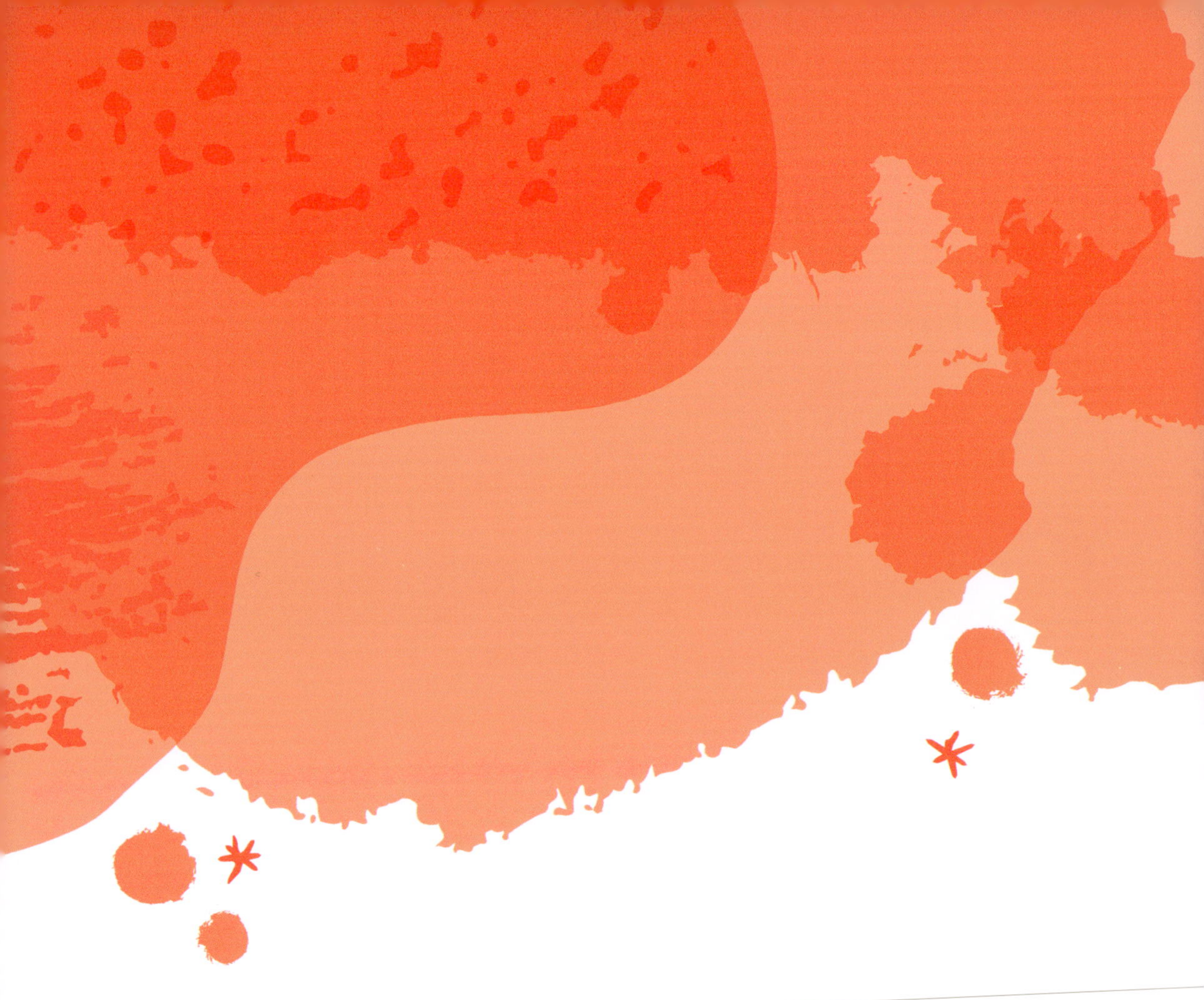

Say hello to zingers.

Intense nerve pain
is another unwelcome surprise.

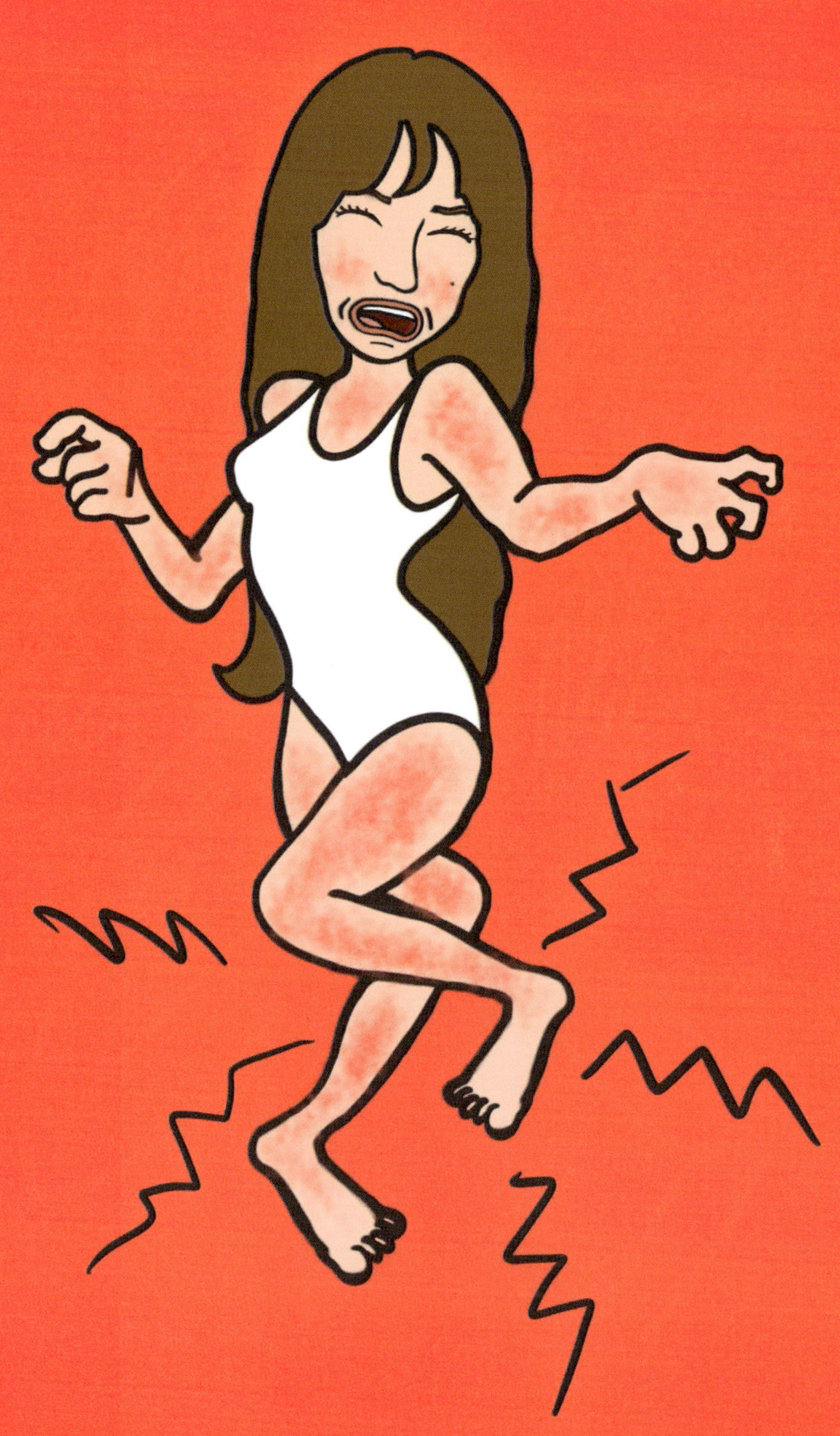

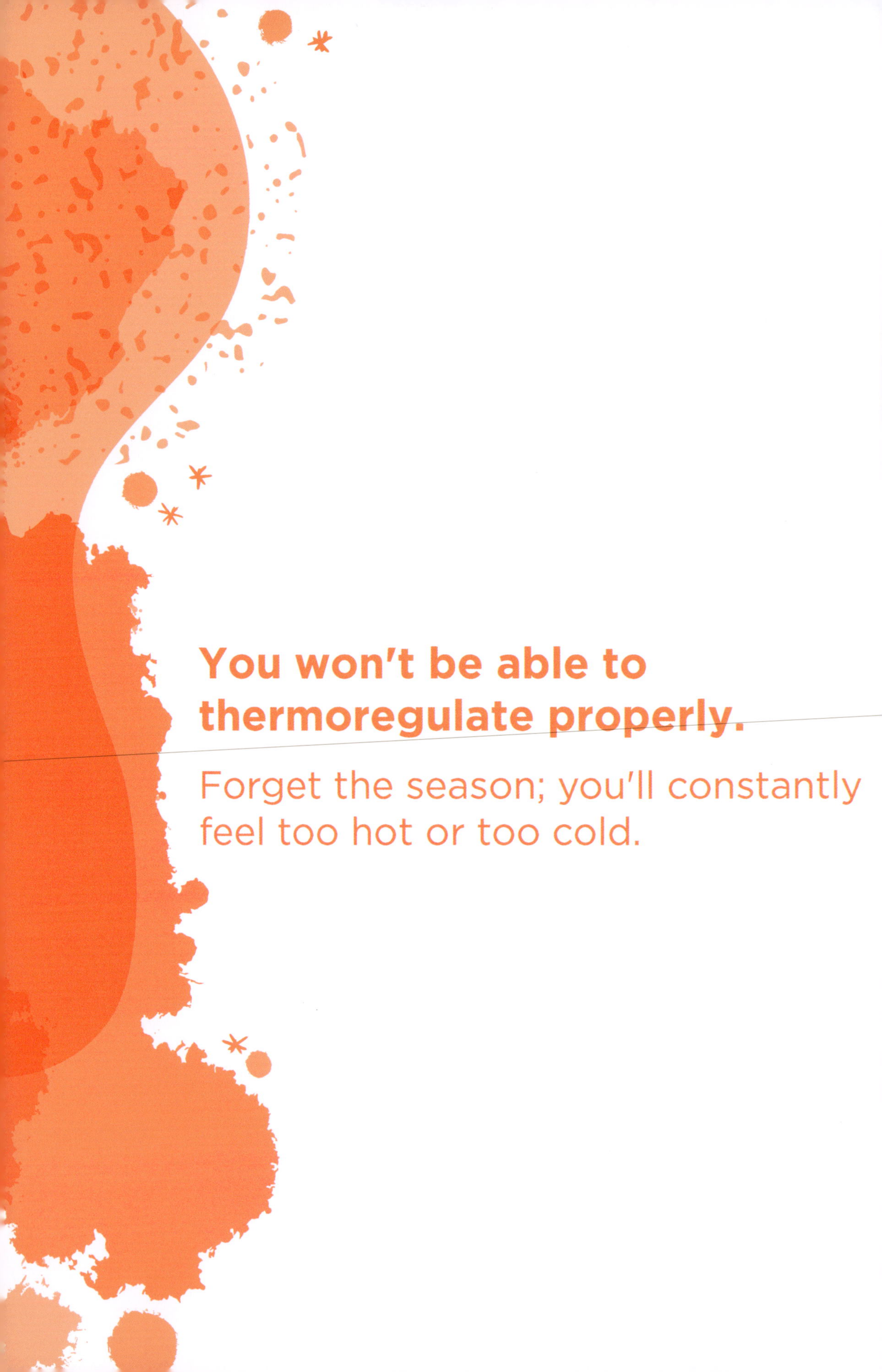

You won't be able to thermoregulate properly.

Forget the season; you'll constantly feel too hot or too cold.

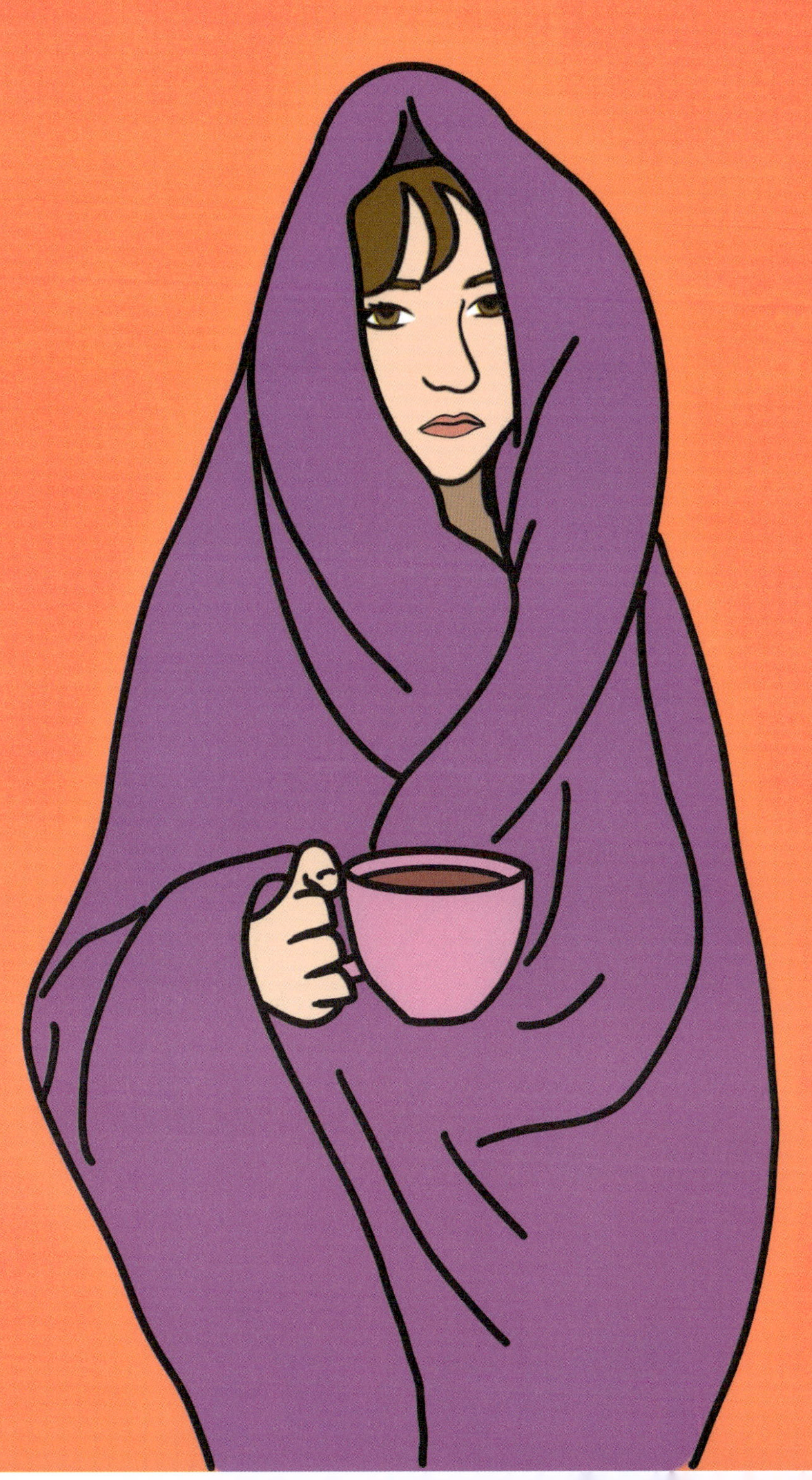

You will spend hundreds of hours researching the condition.....

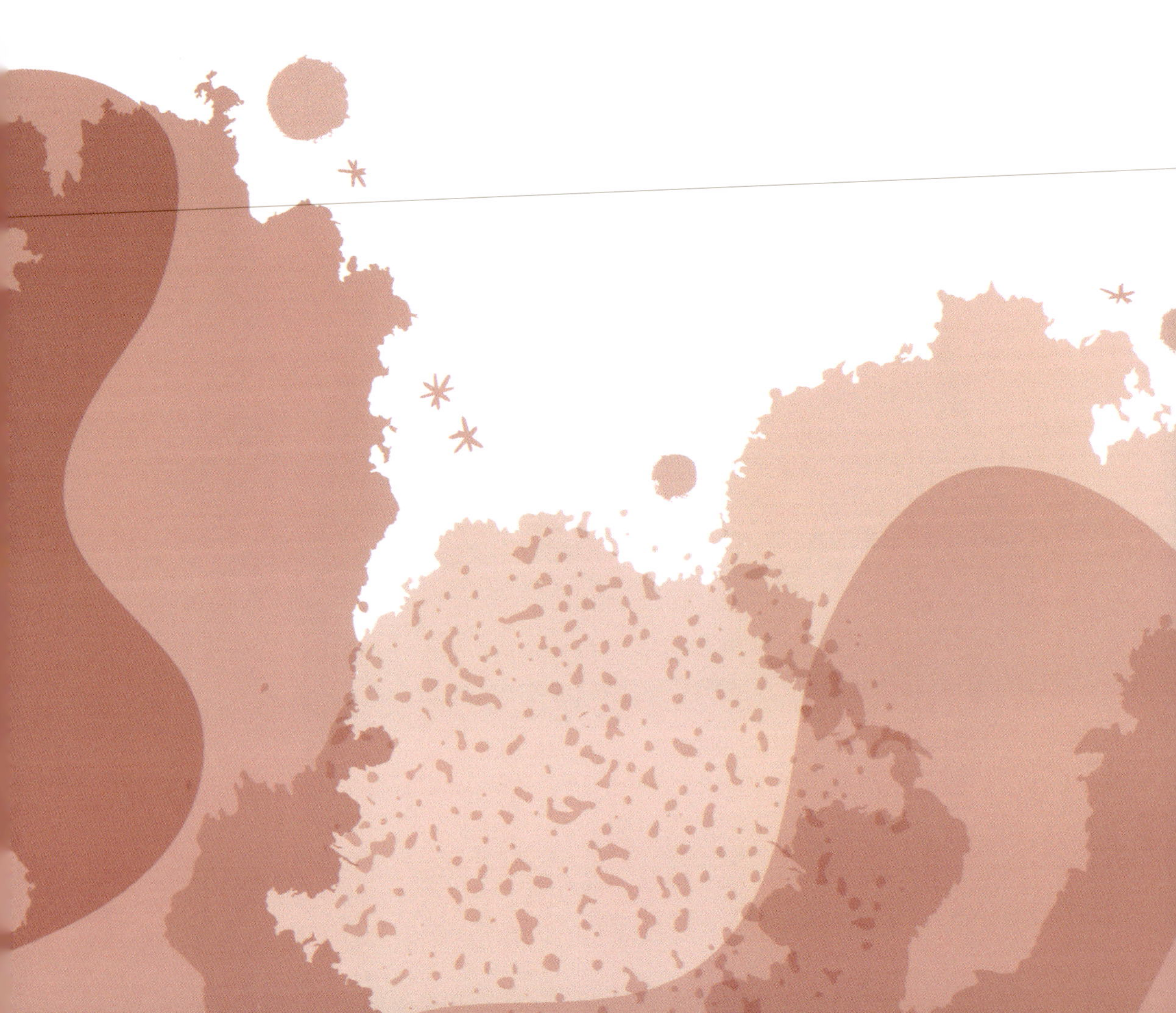

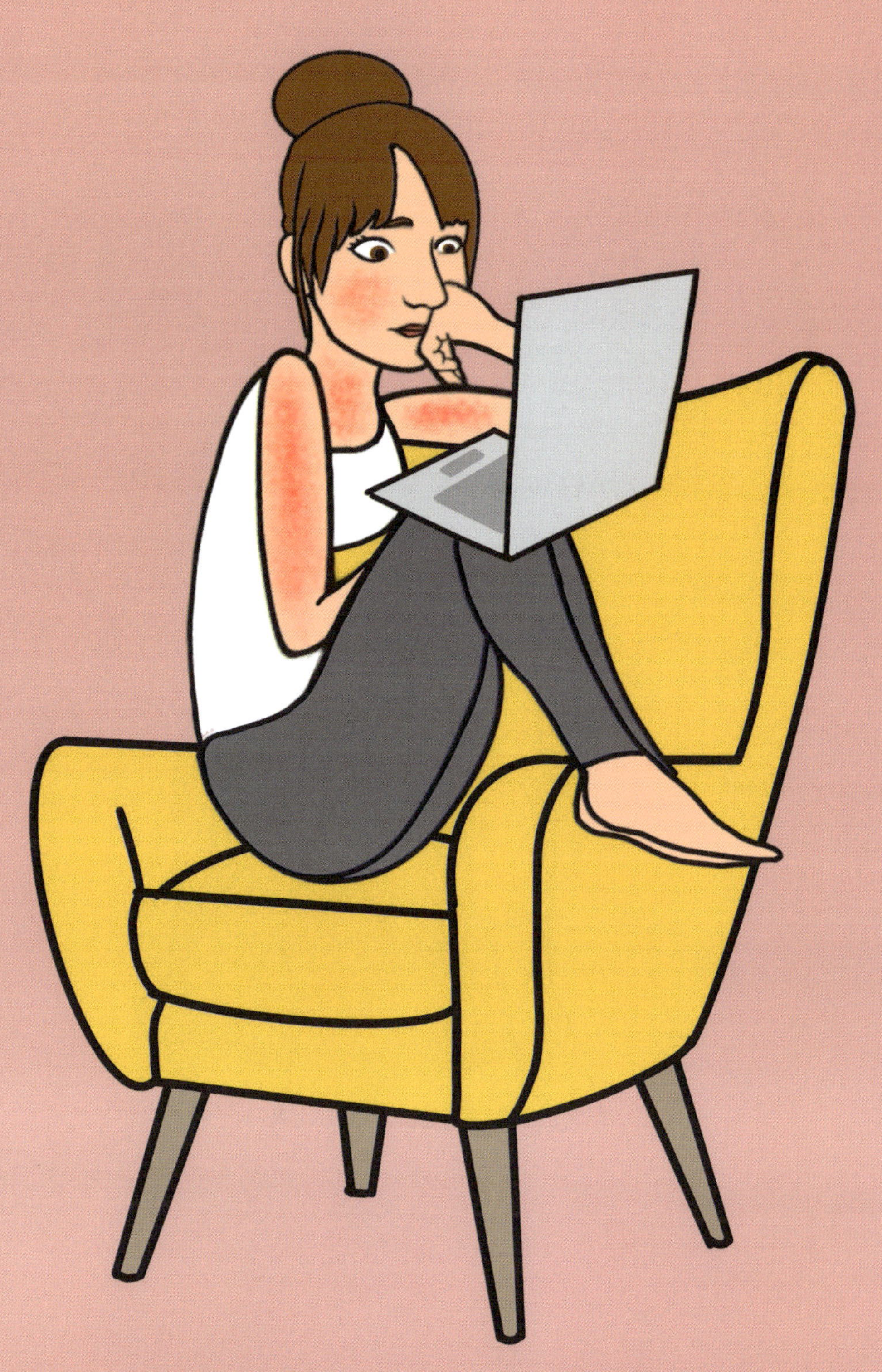

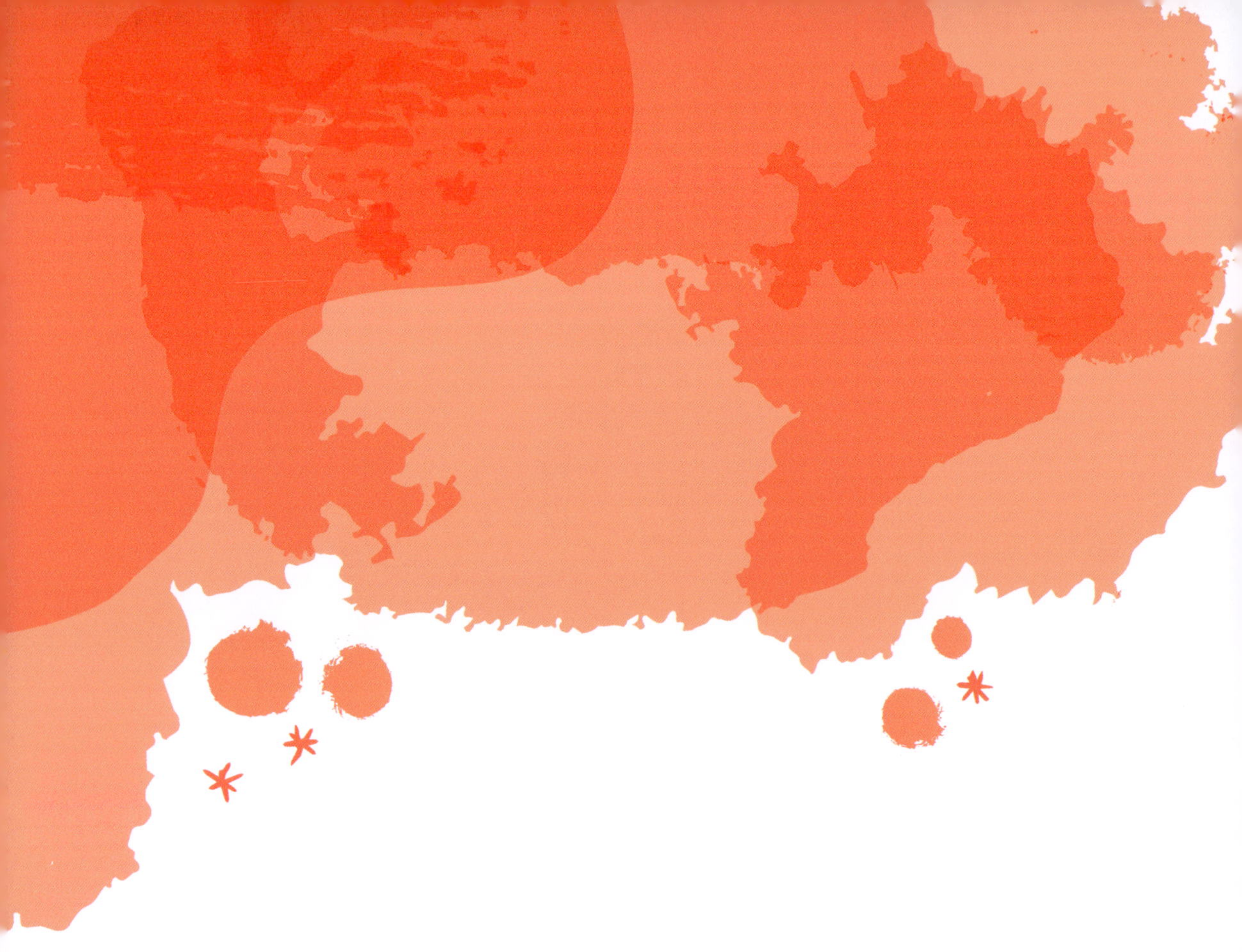

...discovering lots of new acronyms.

Some may change your world.

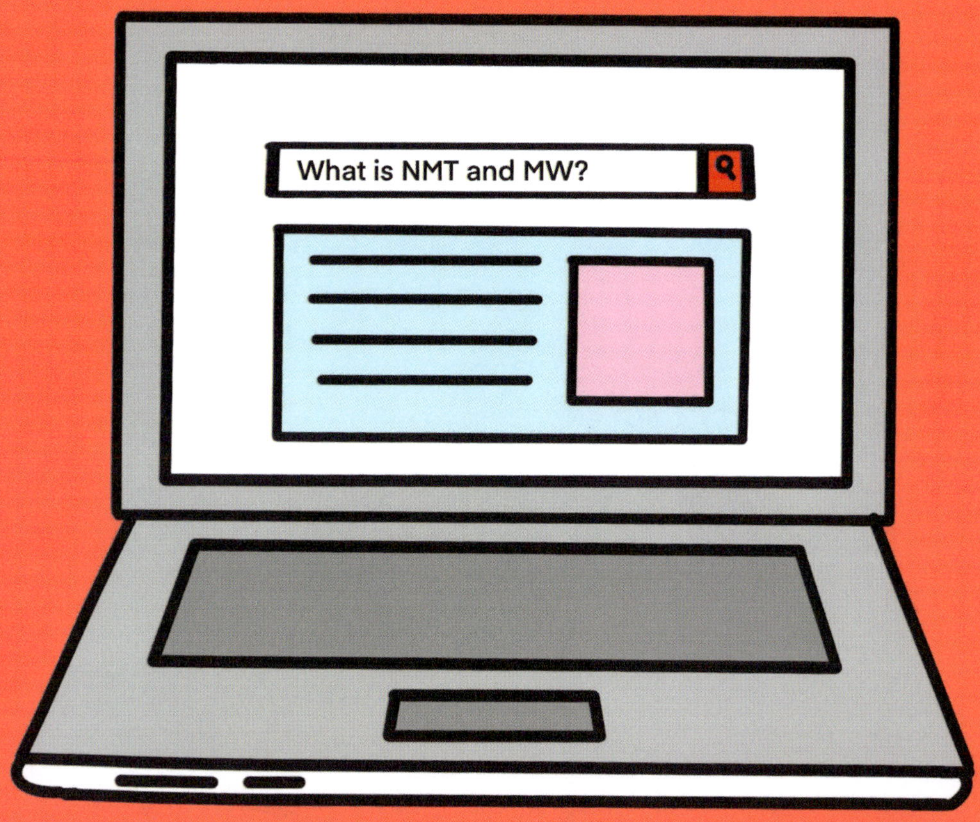
What is NMT and MW?

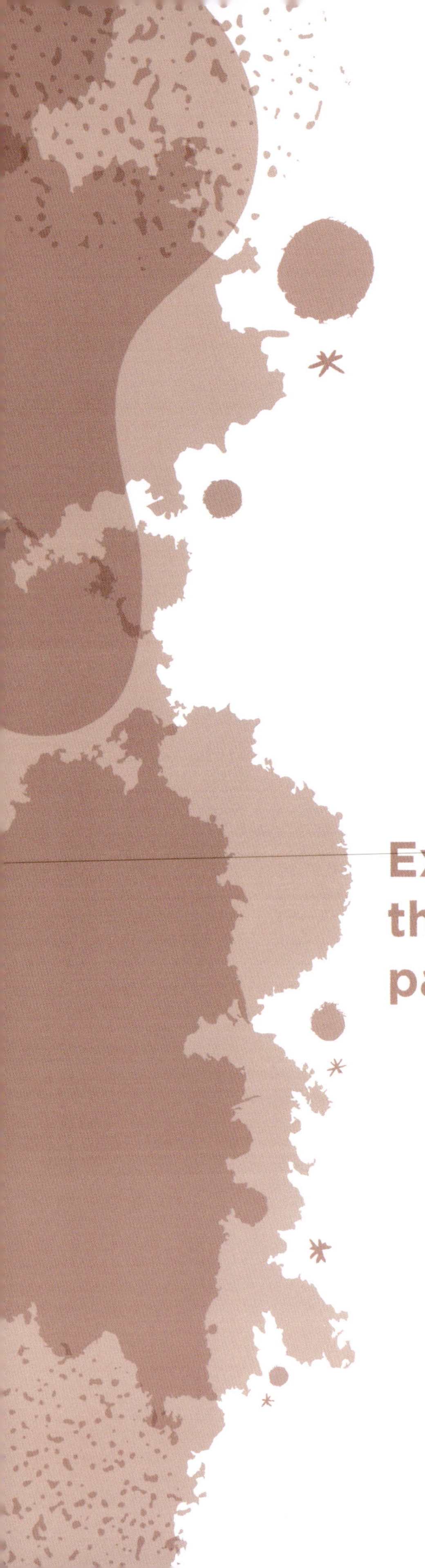

Exploring alternative therapies becomes part of the journey.

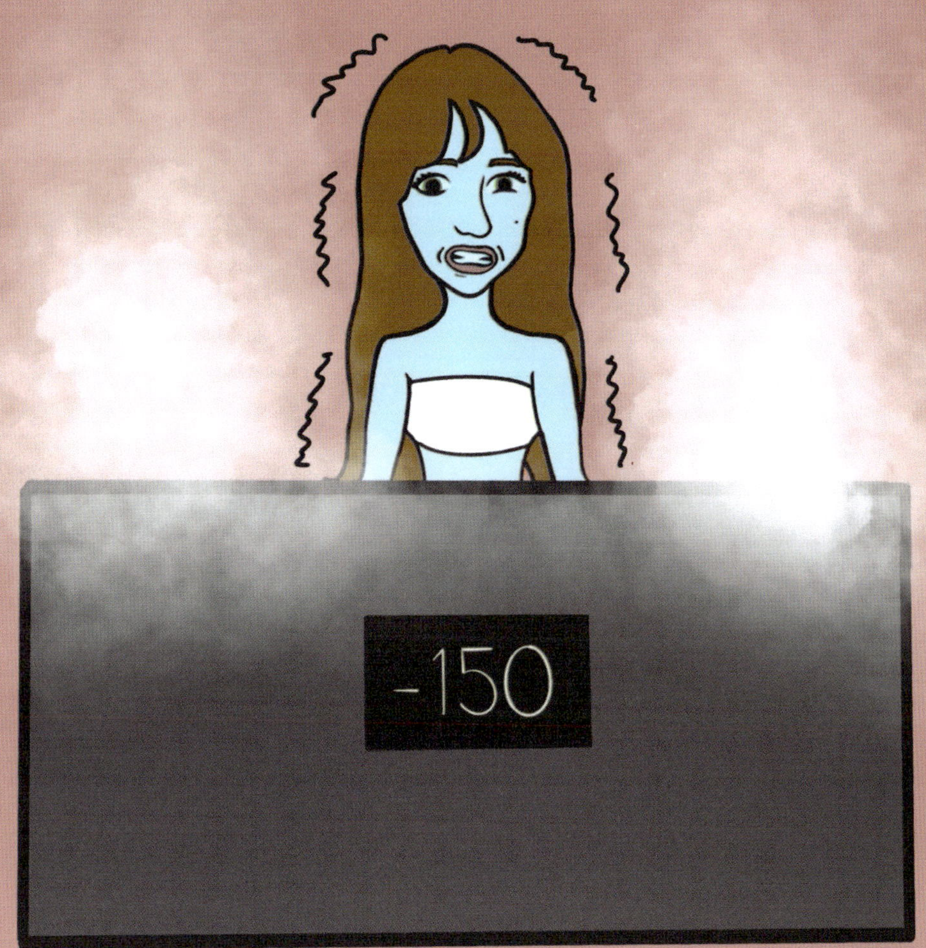
-150

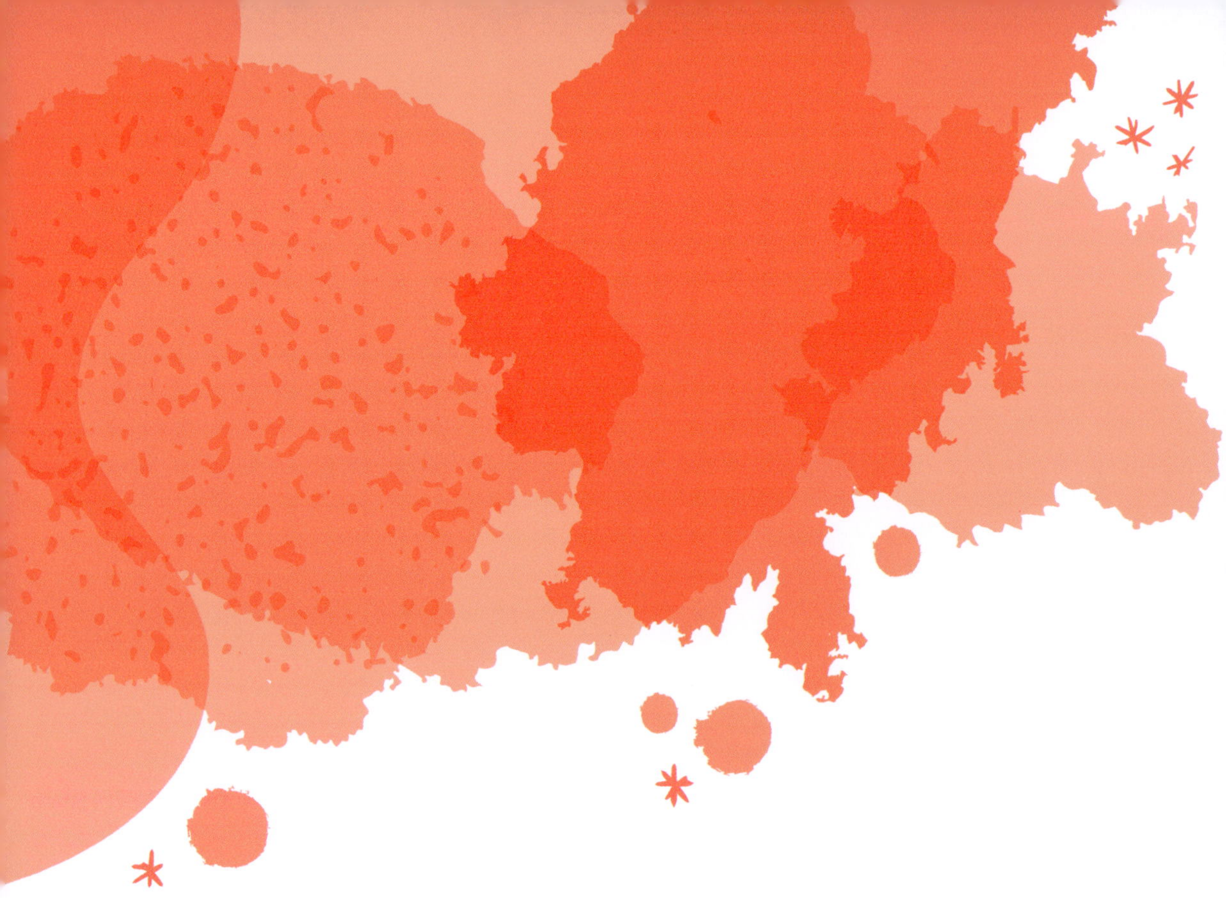

Swollen lymph nodes come and go.

You'll be surprised how many different places these can swell.

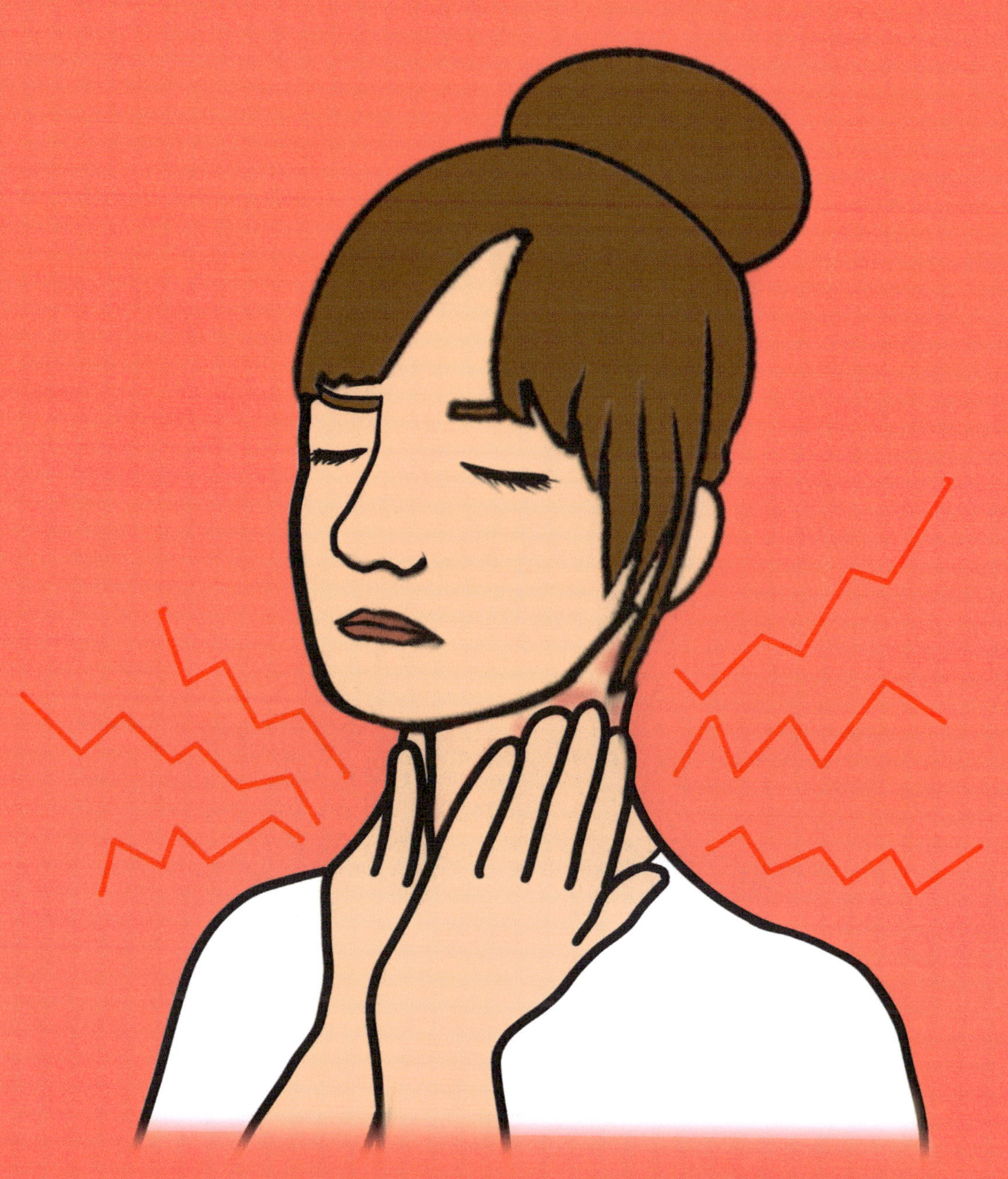

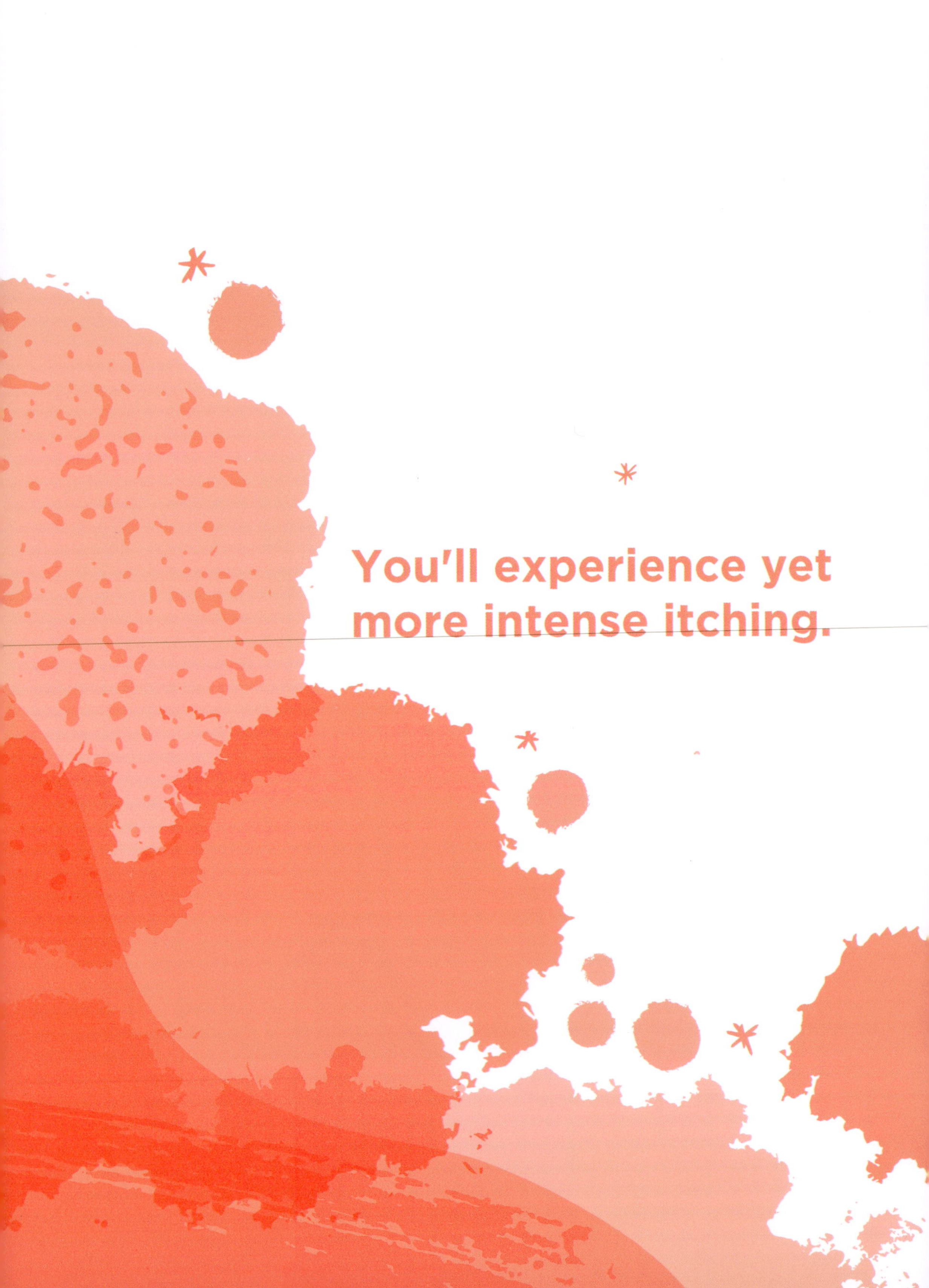

You'll experience yet more intense itching.

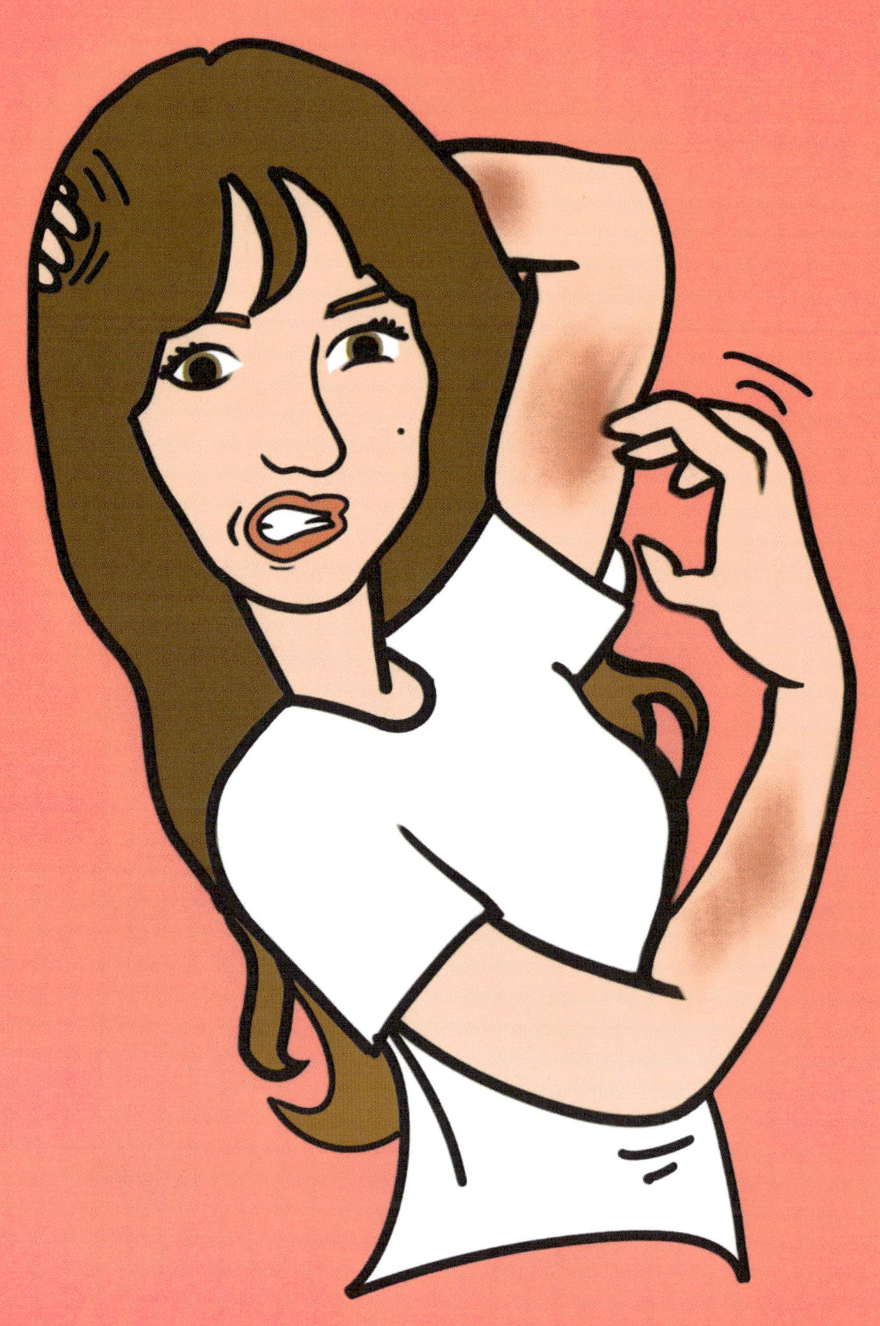

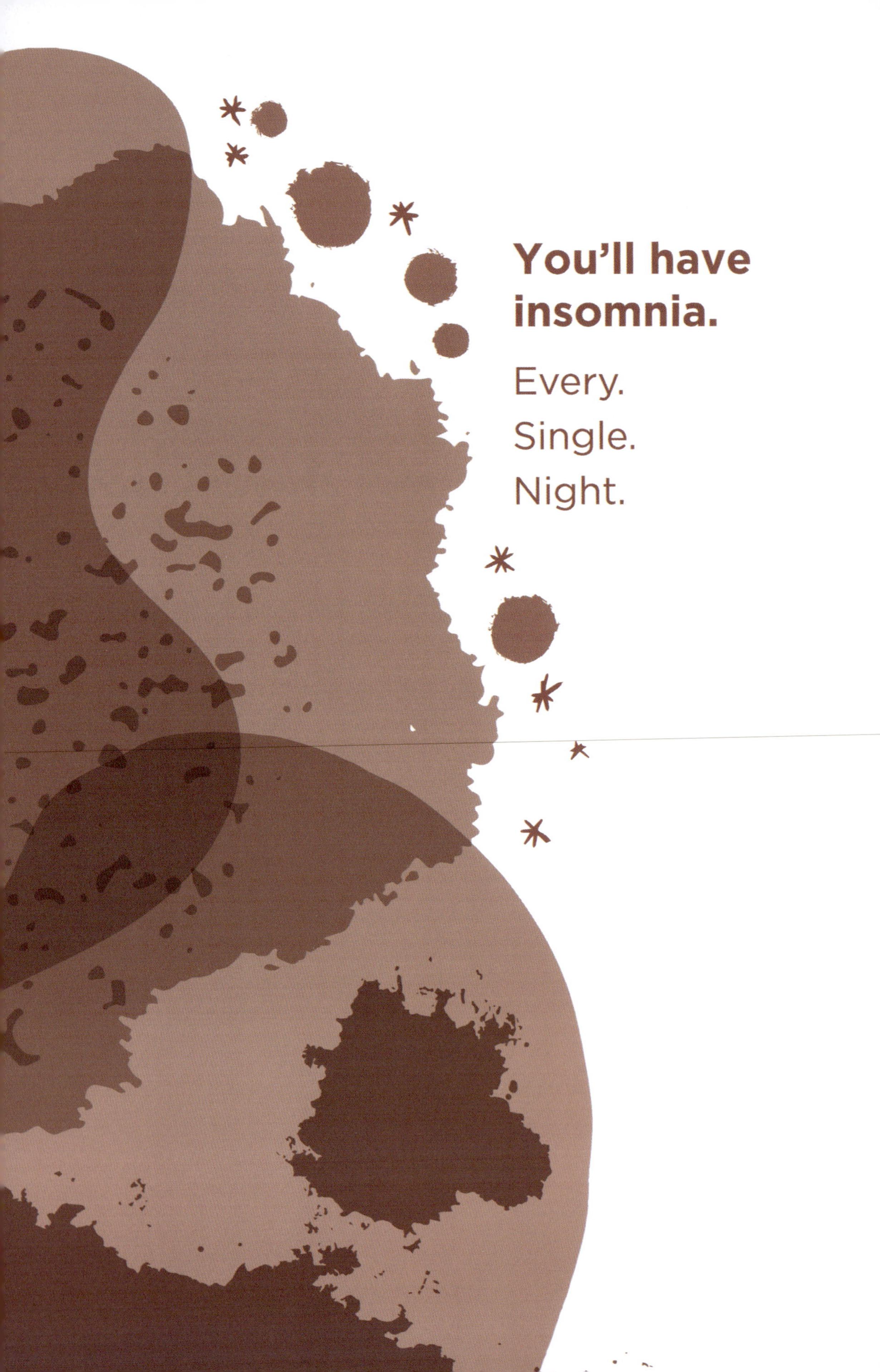

You'll have insomnia.

Every.

Single.

Night.

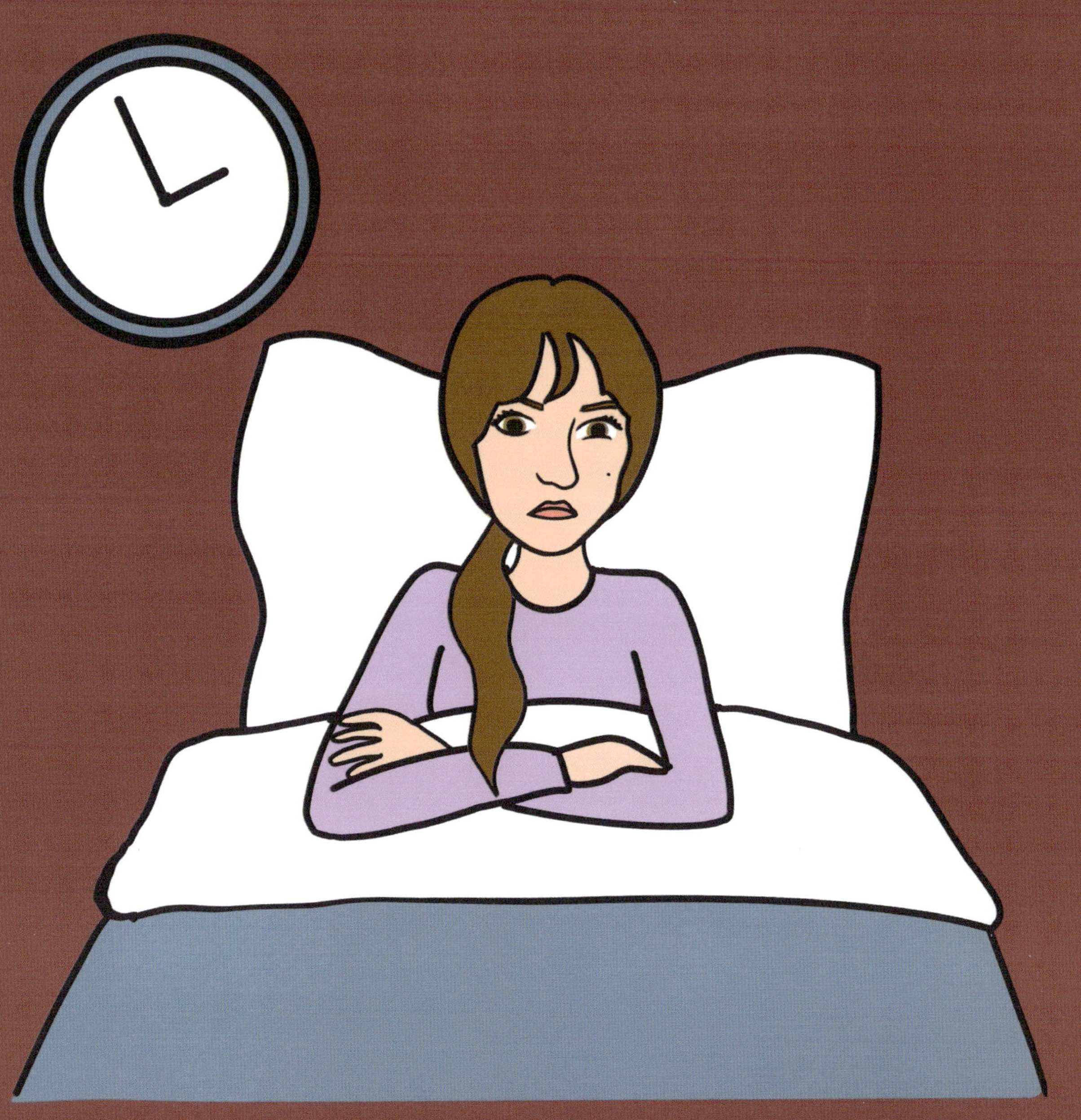

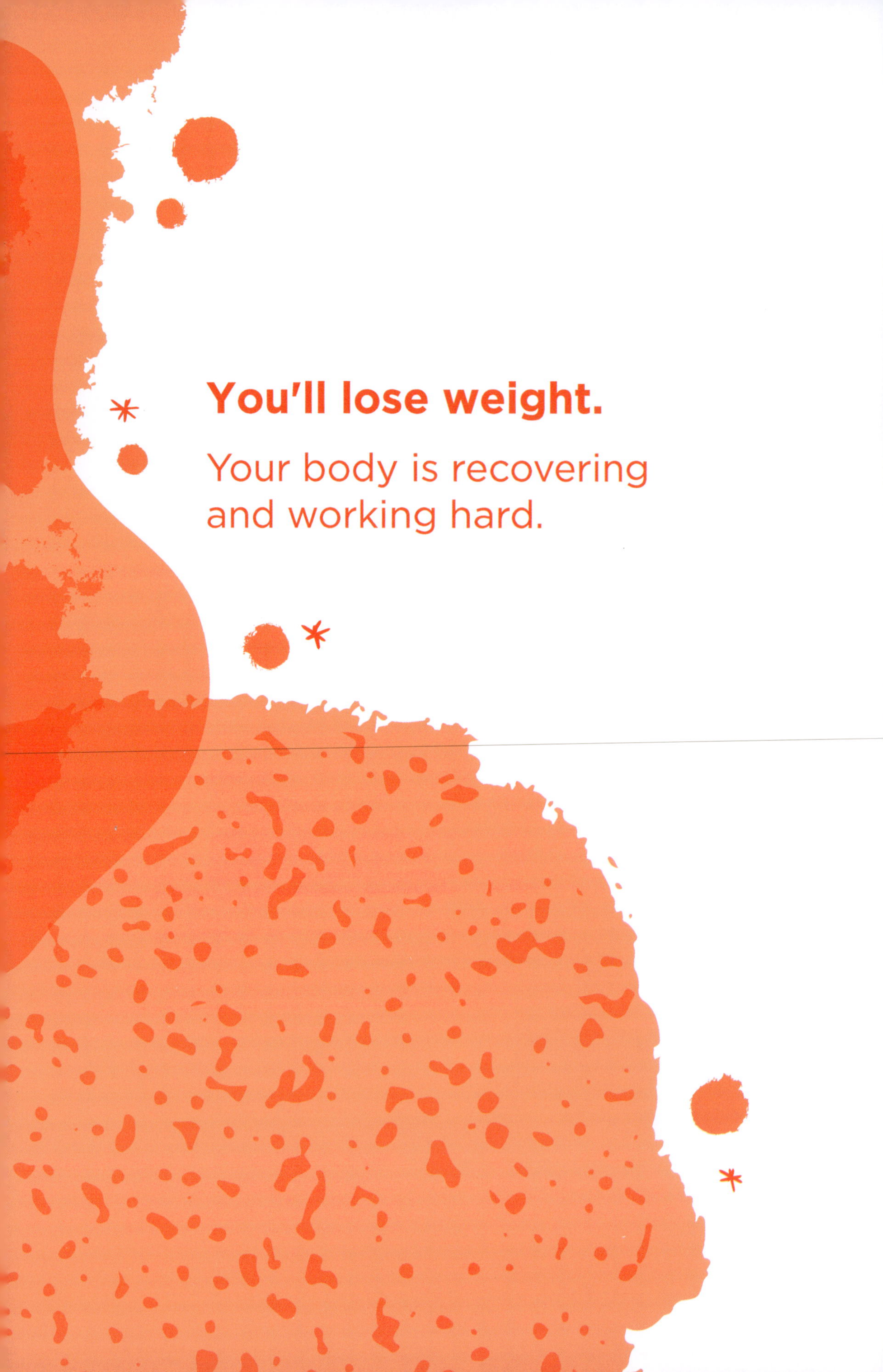

You'll lose weight.

Your body is recovering and working hard.

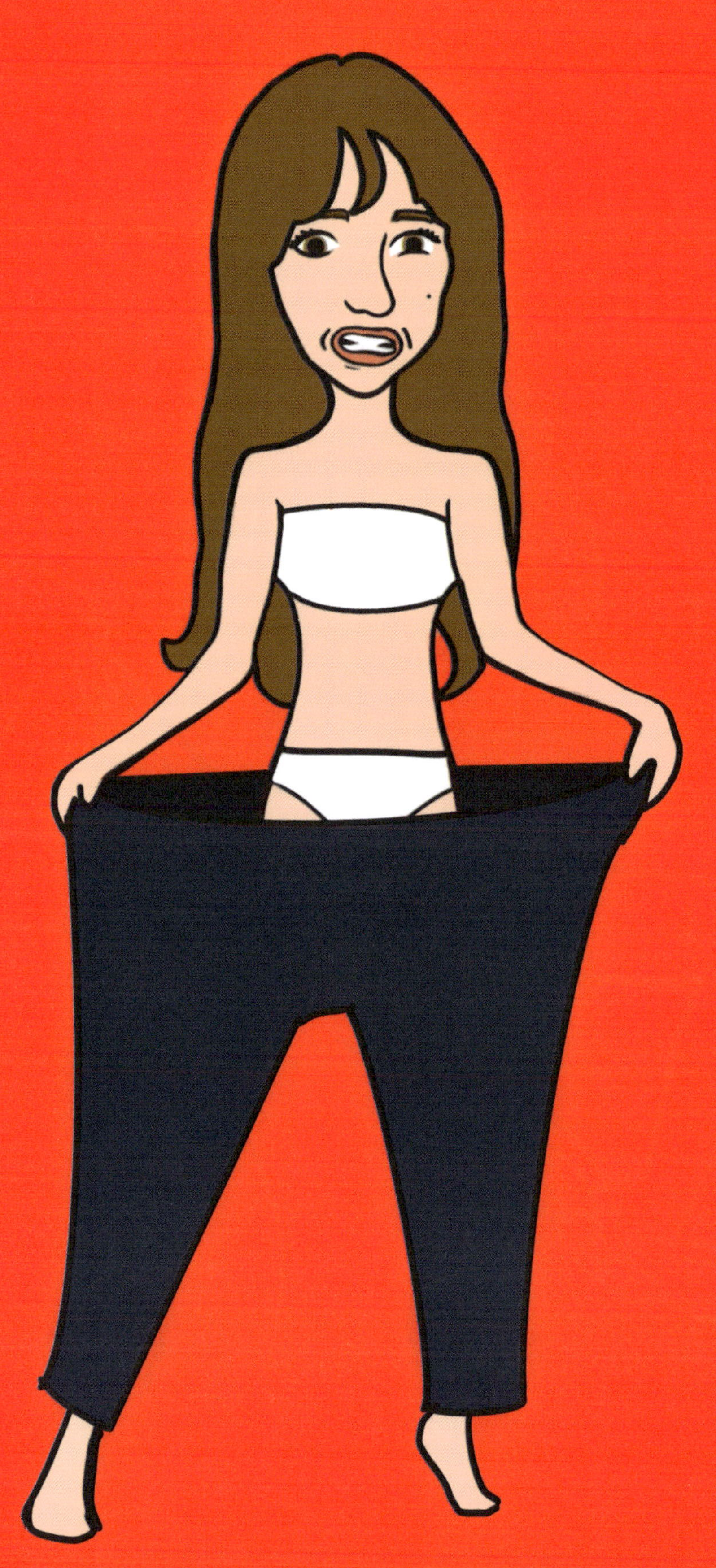

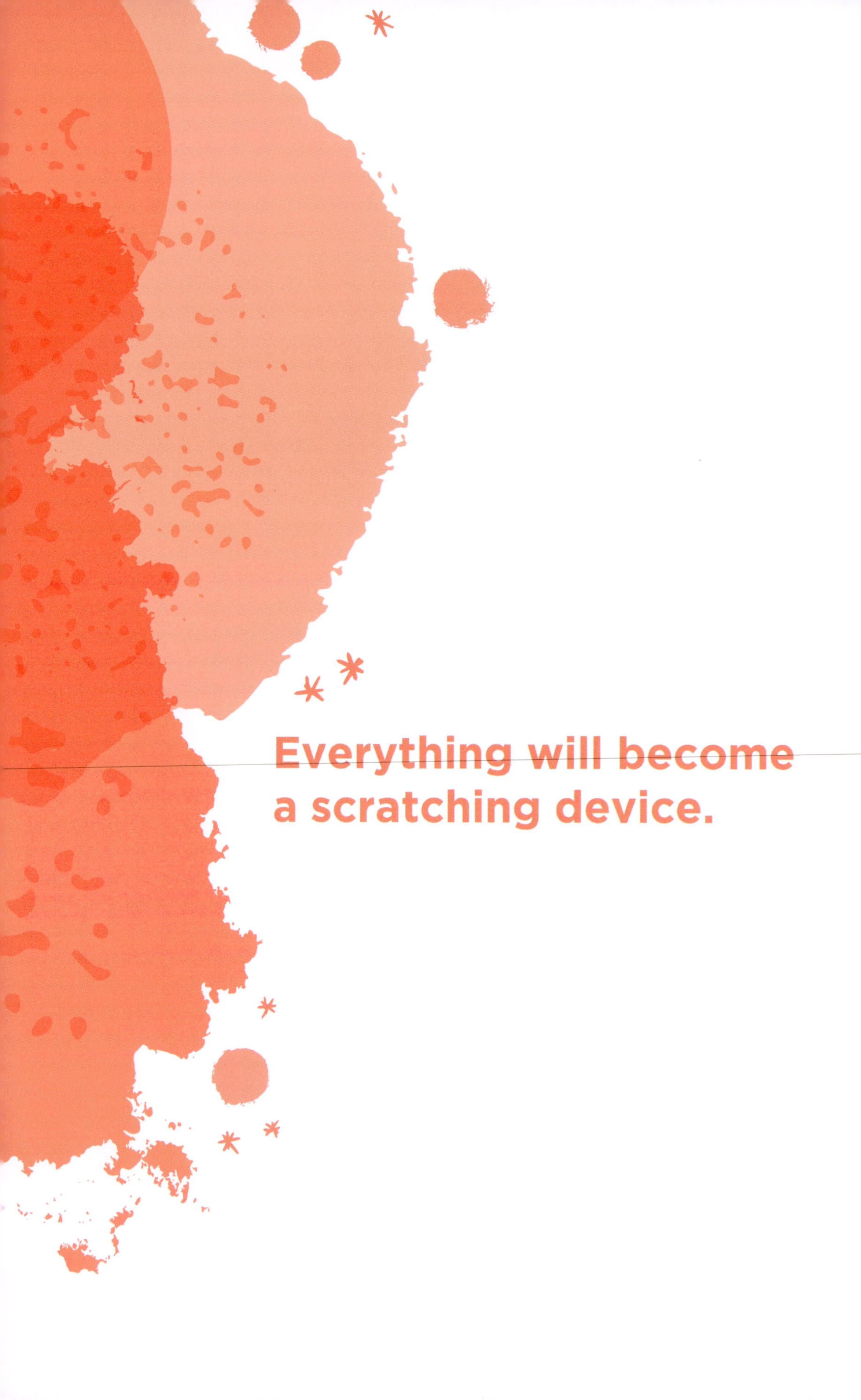

Everything will become
a scratching device.

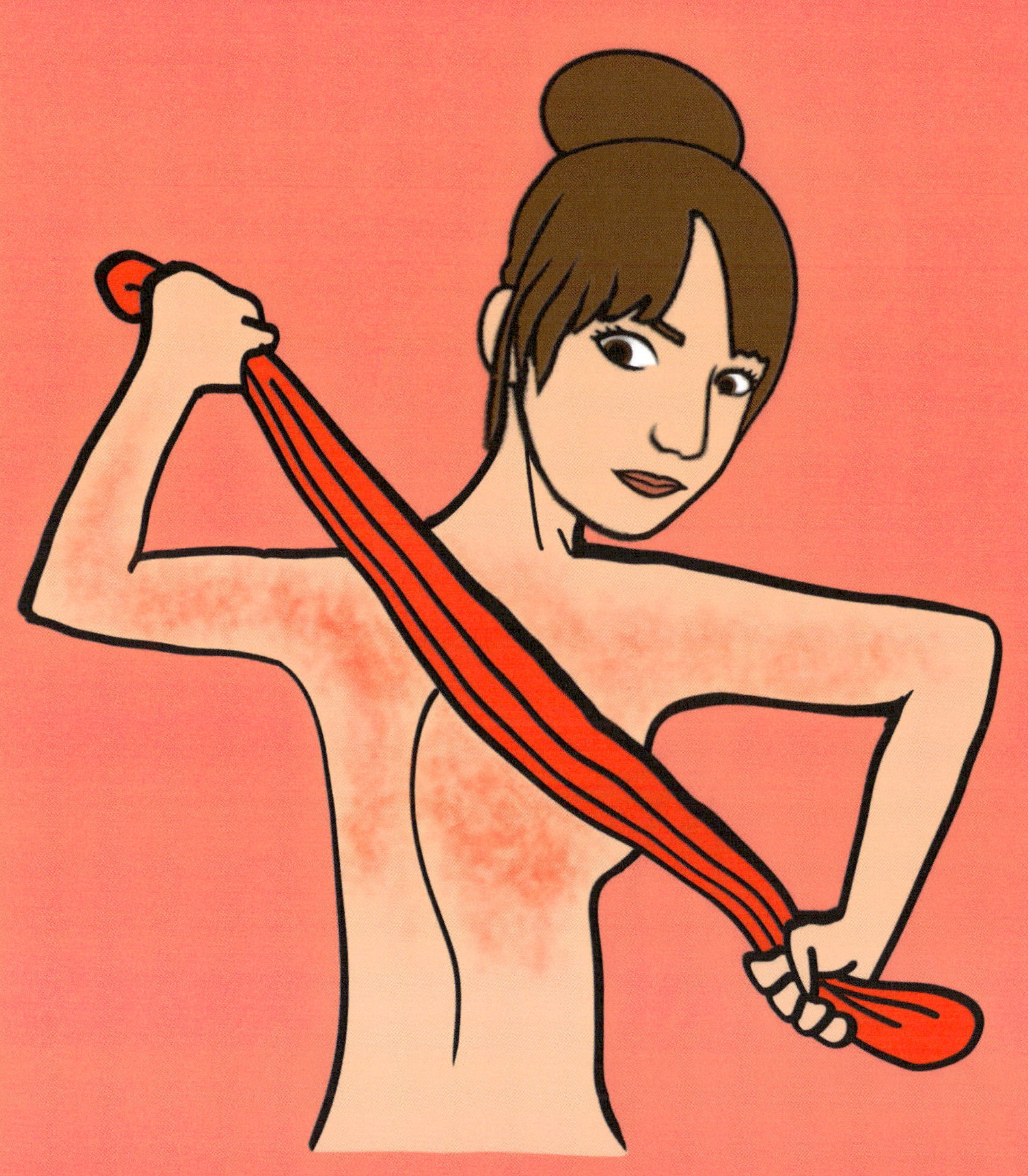

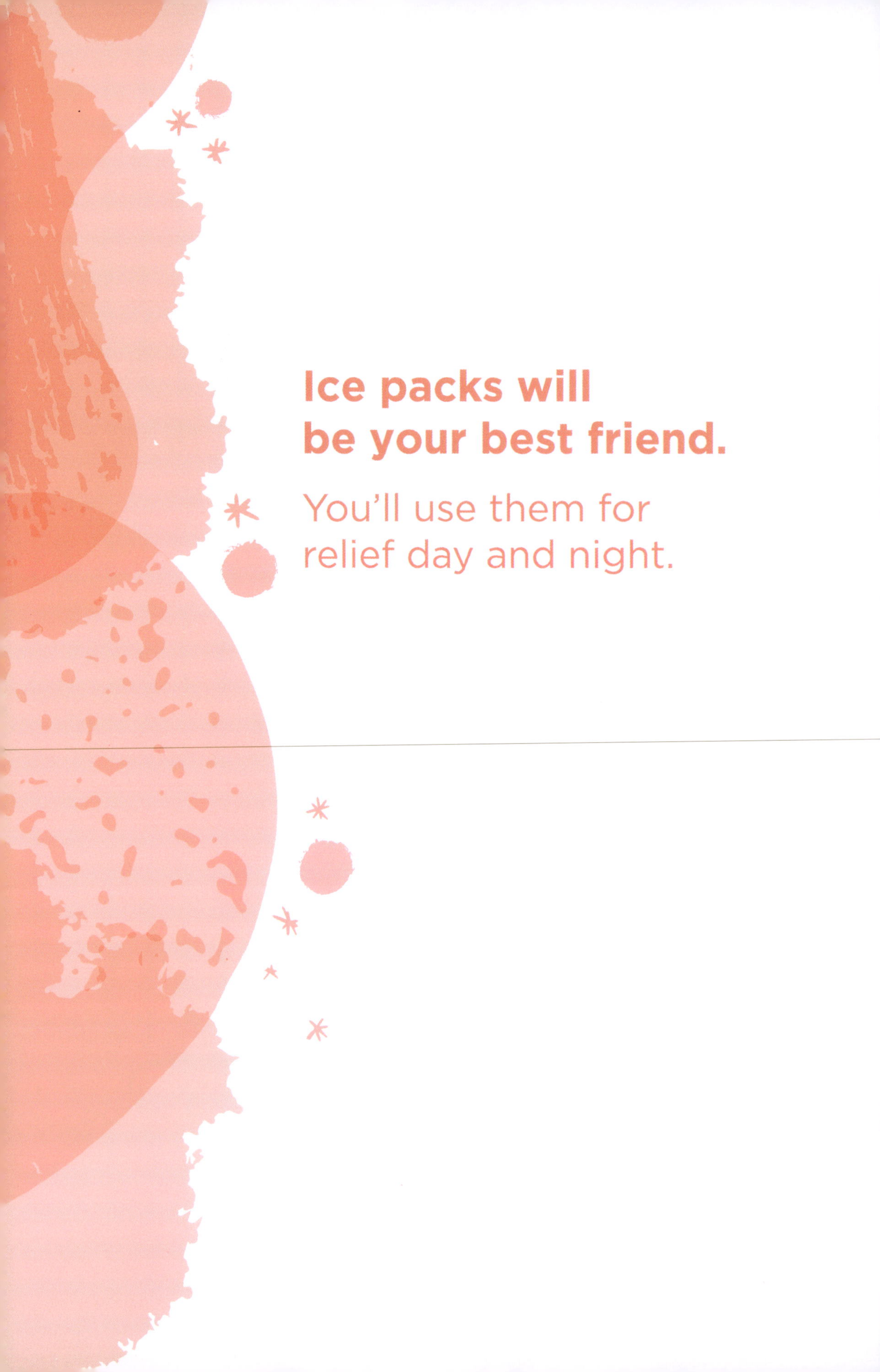

Ice packs will be your best friend.

You'll use them for relief day and night.

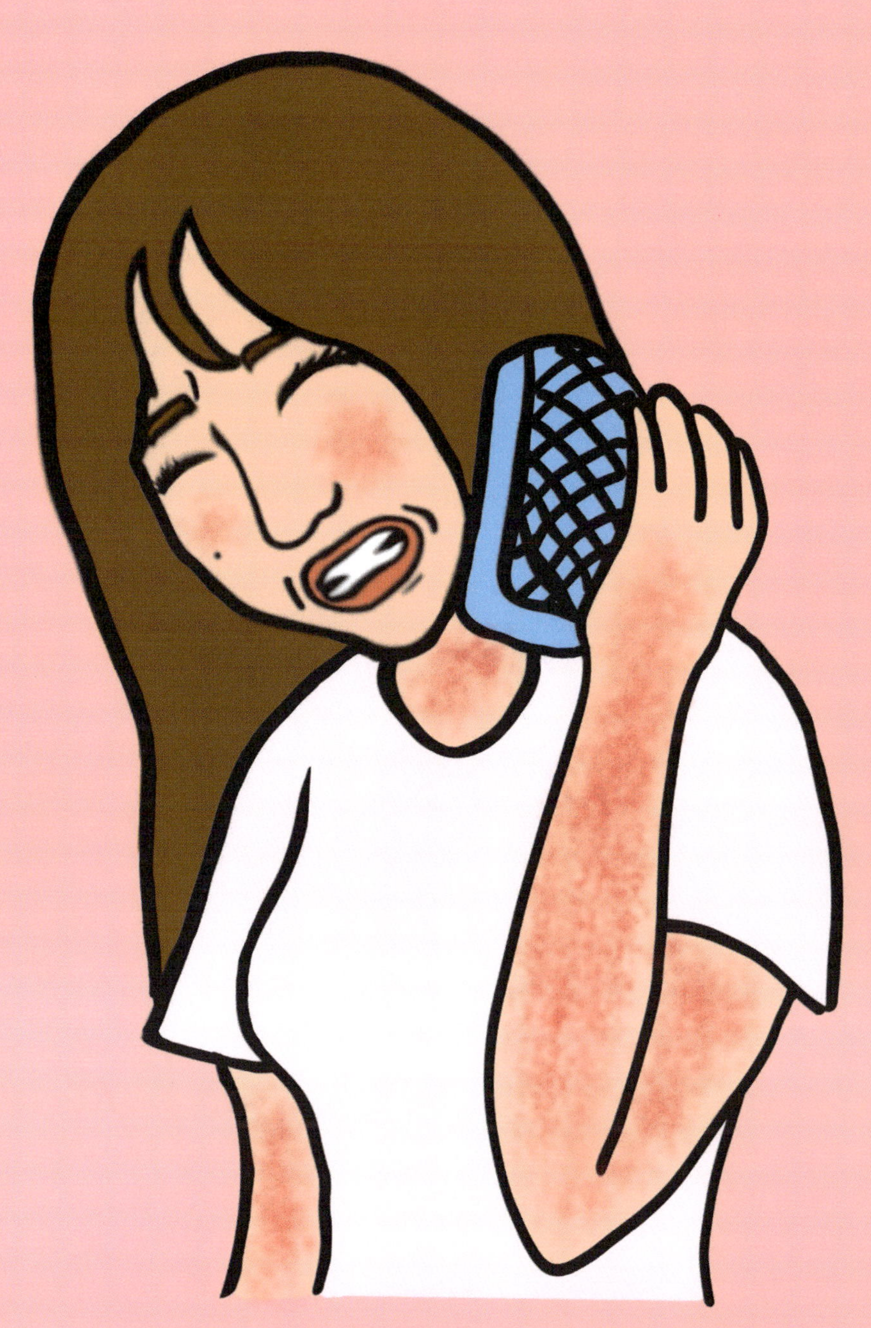

Your nails will change.

You'll discover that fake nails damage your skin less when scratching.

Who'd have thought?

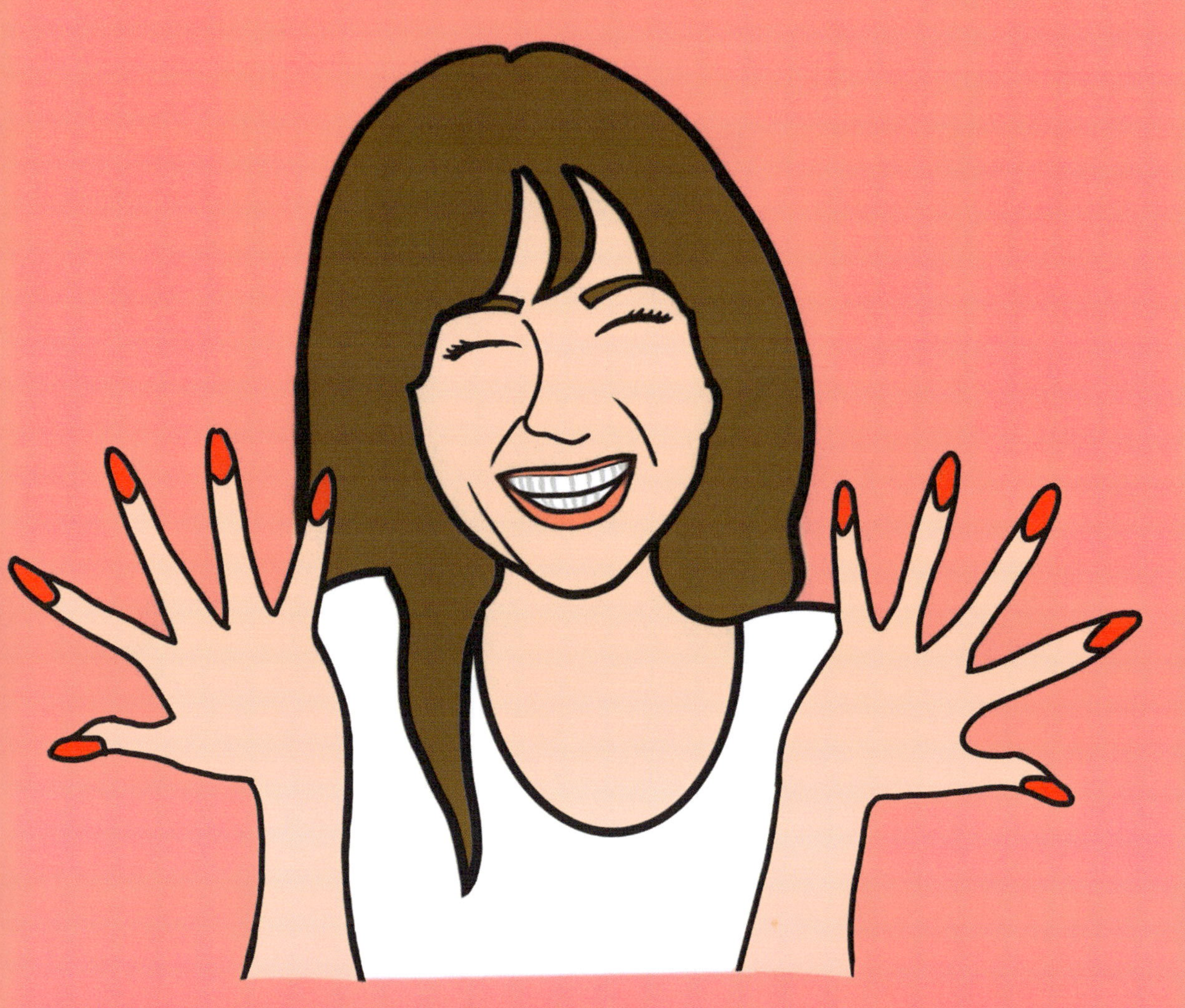

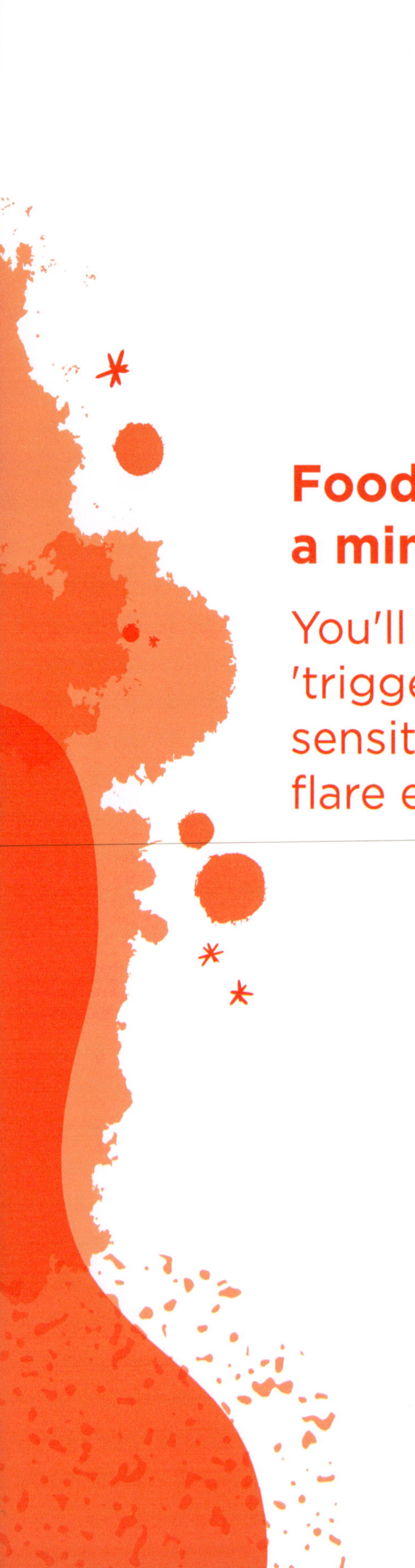

Food will become a minefield.

You'll try to eliminate 'trigger foods' so your sensitive skin doesn't flare even more.

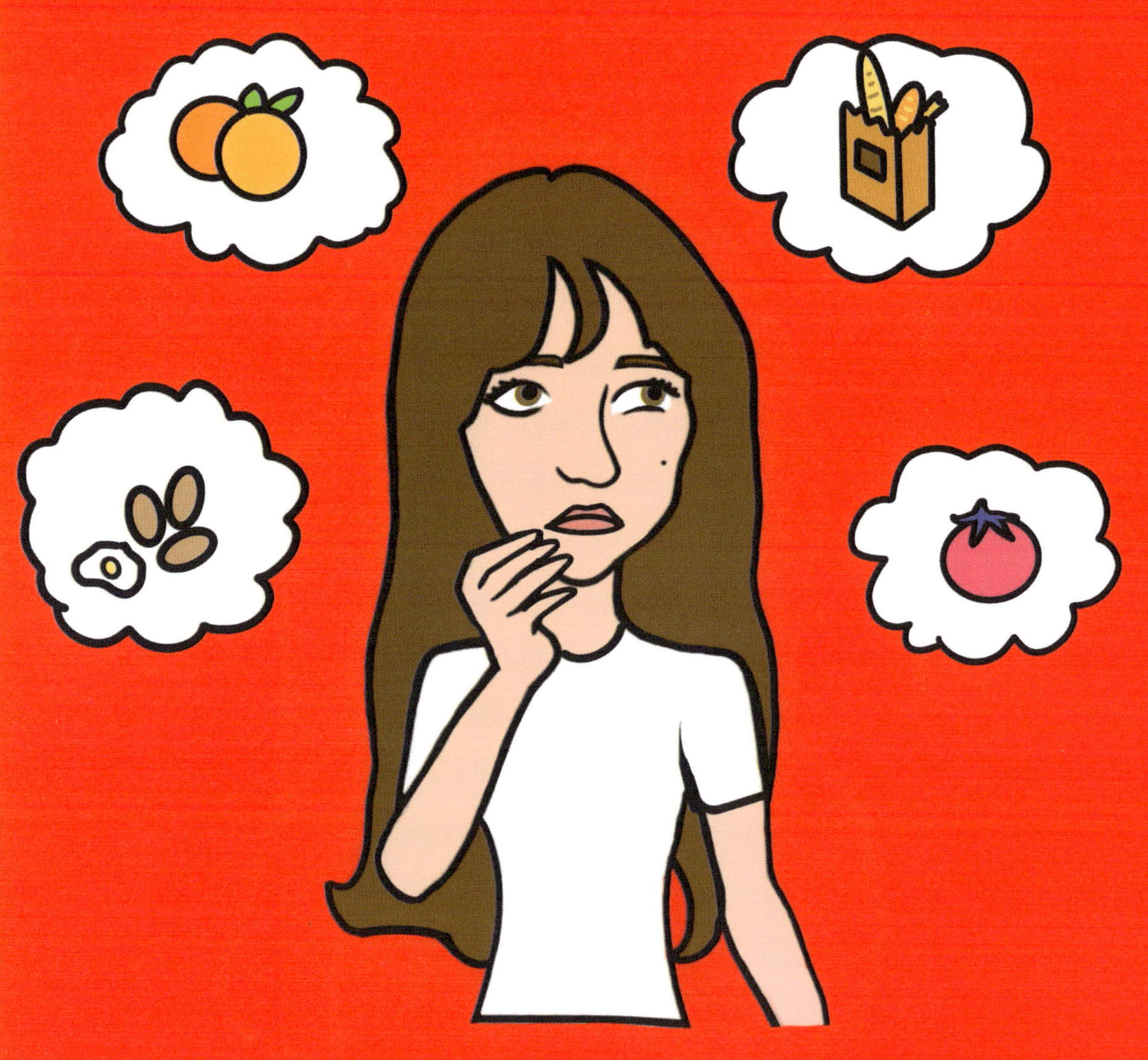

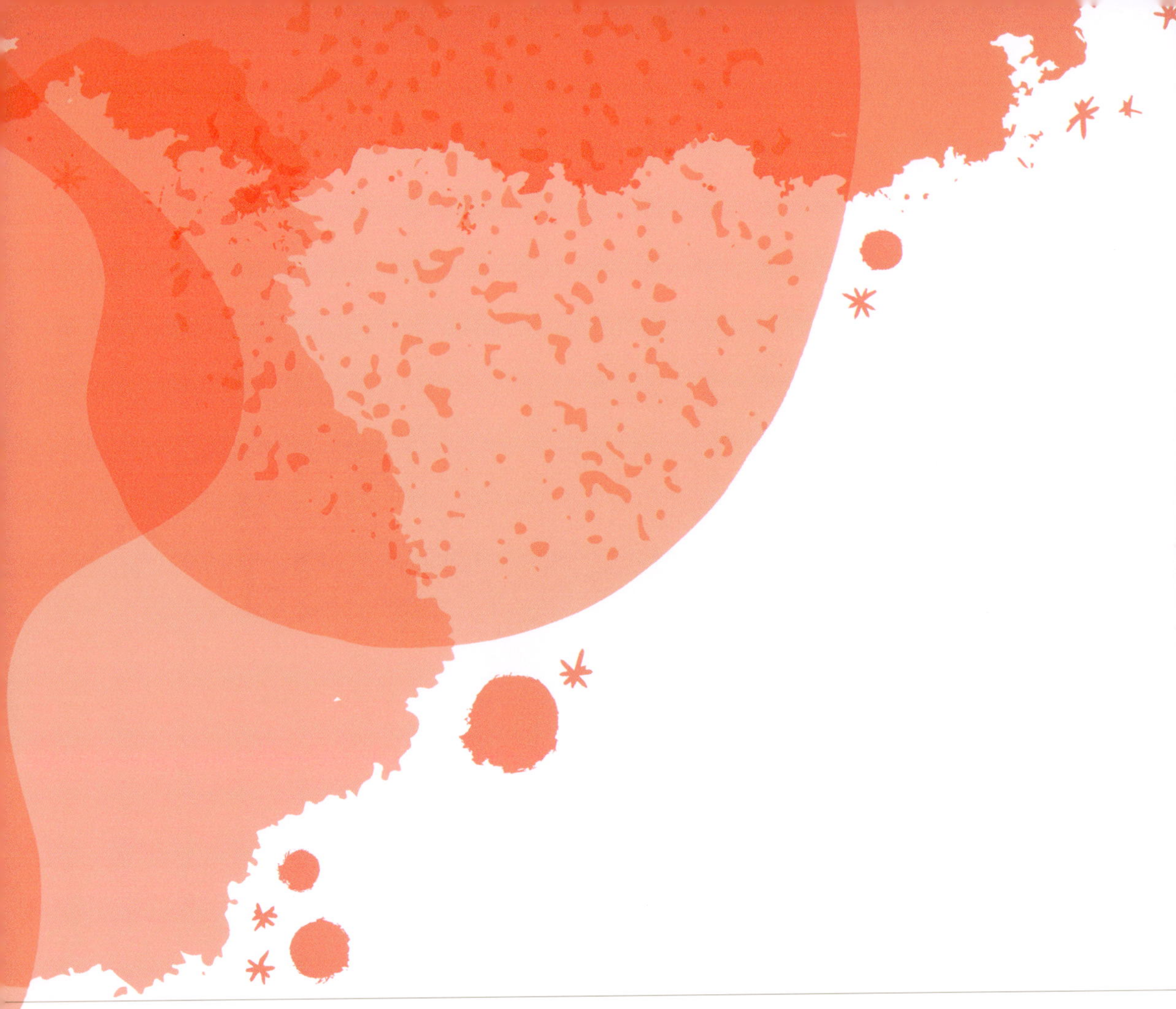

Everything will make you flare.

You'll flare for no reason at all.

It's all part of recovery.

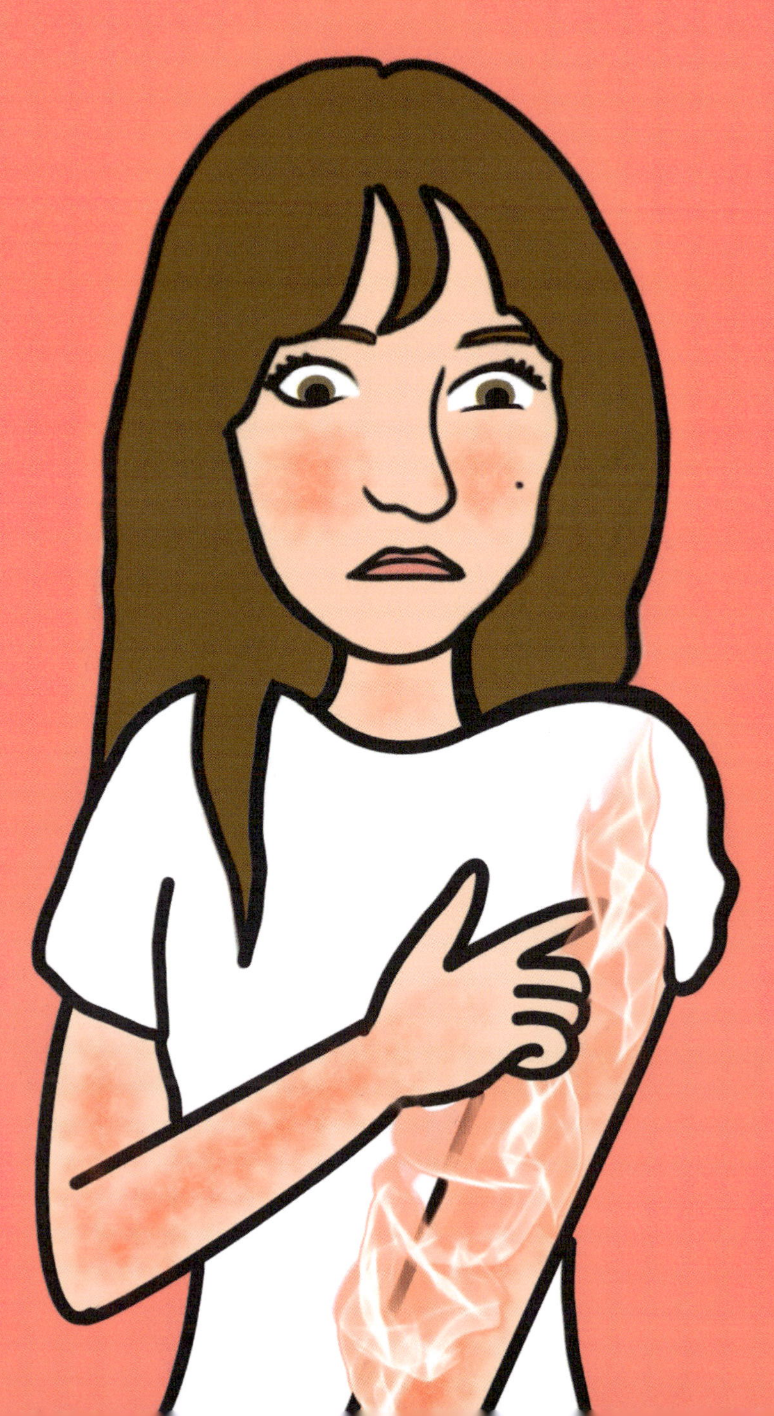

The anxiety can be crippling.

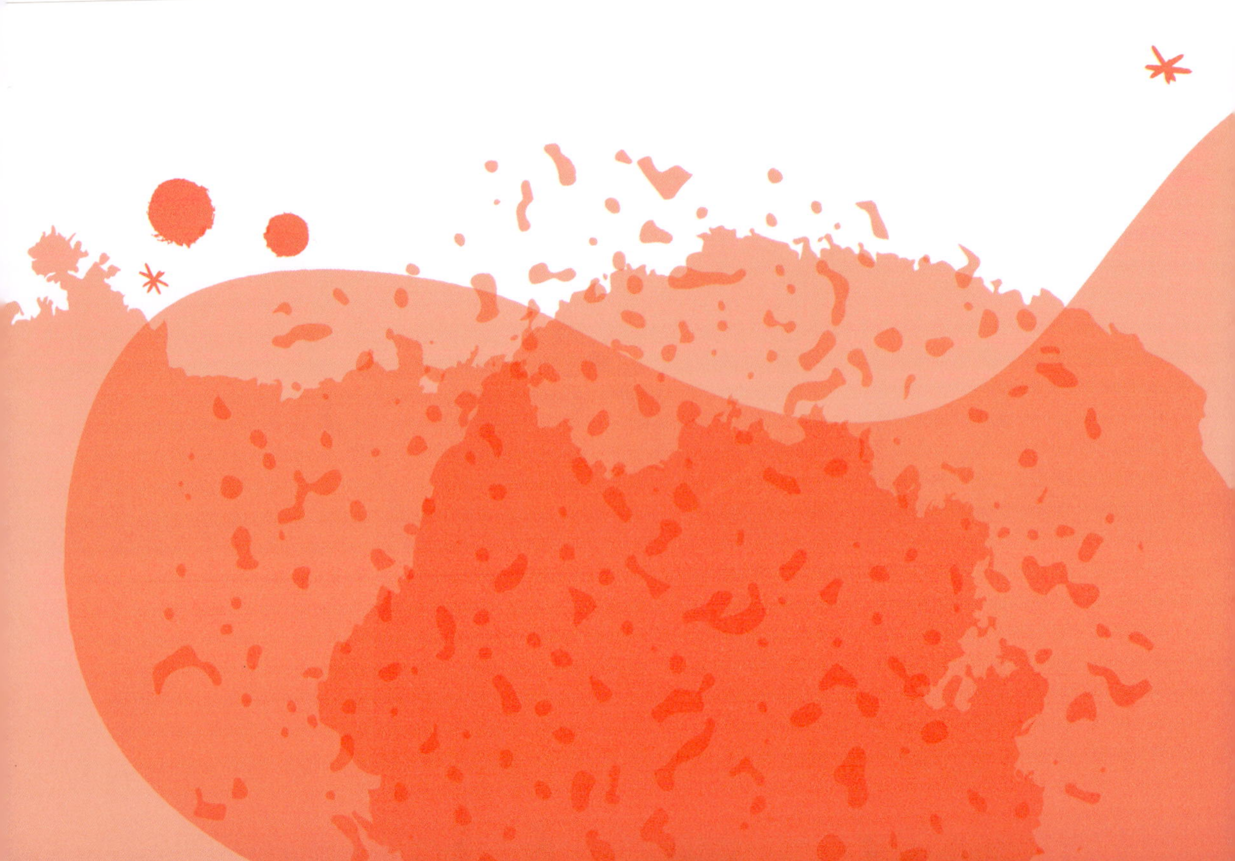

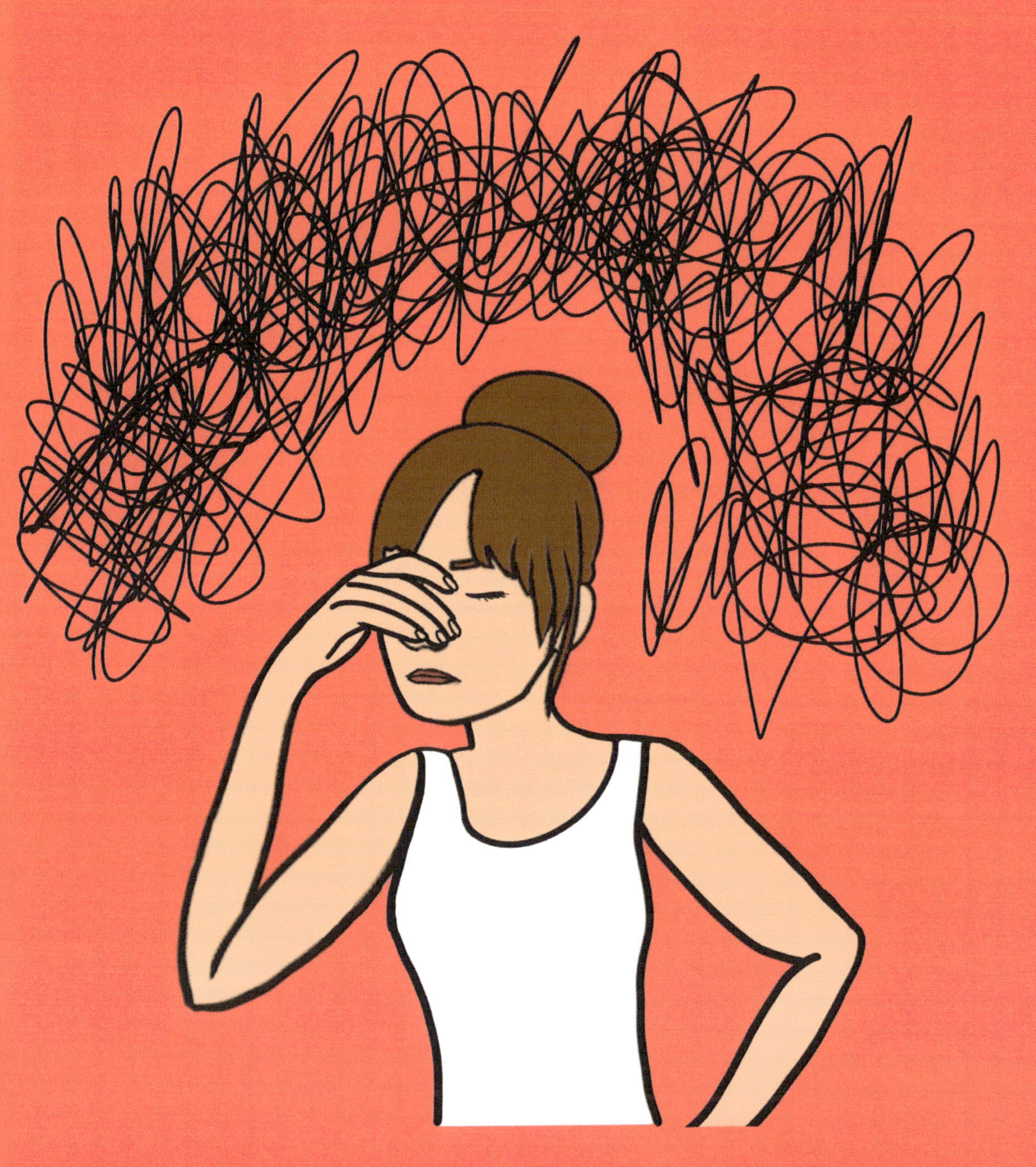

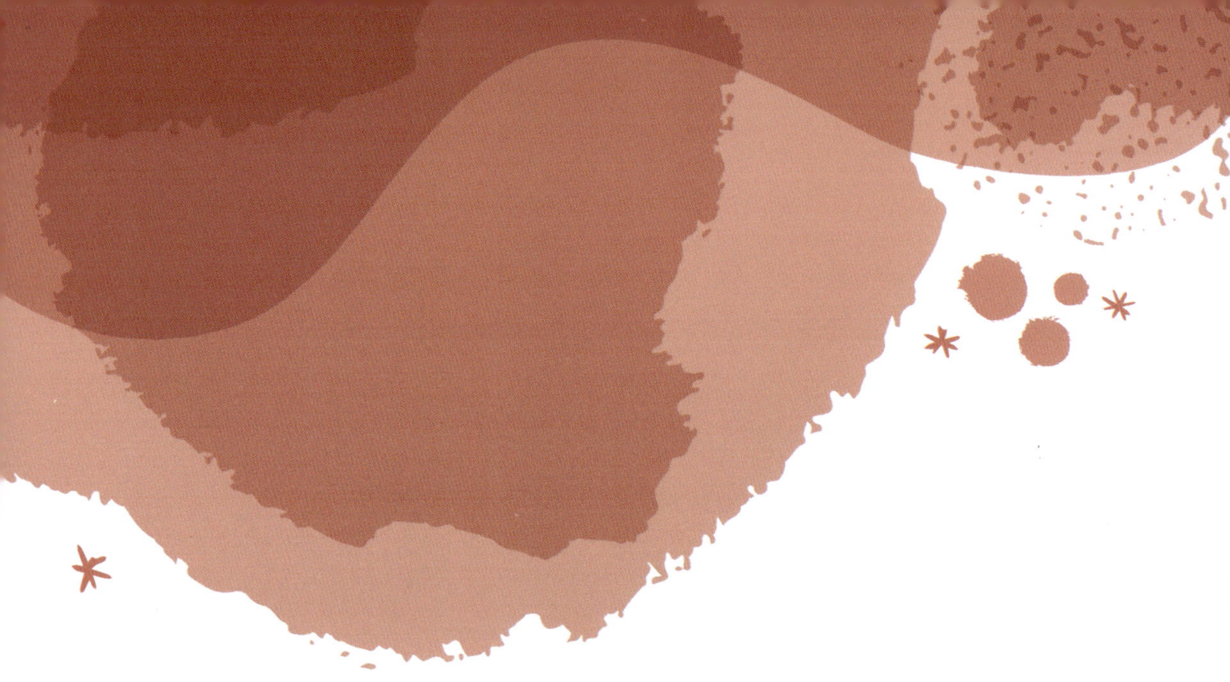

You'll do lots of record keeping.

Although you don't want to take photos, you'll be so glad you did when you see how far you've come.

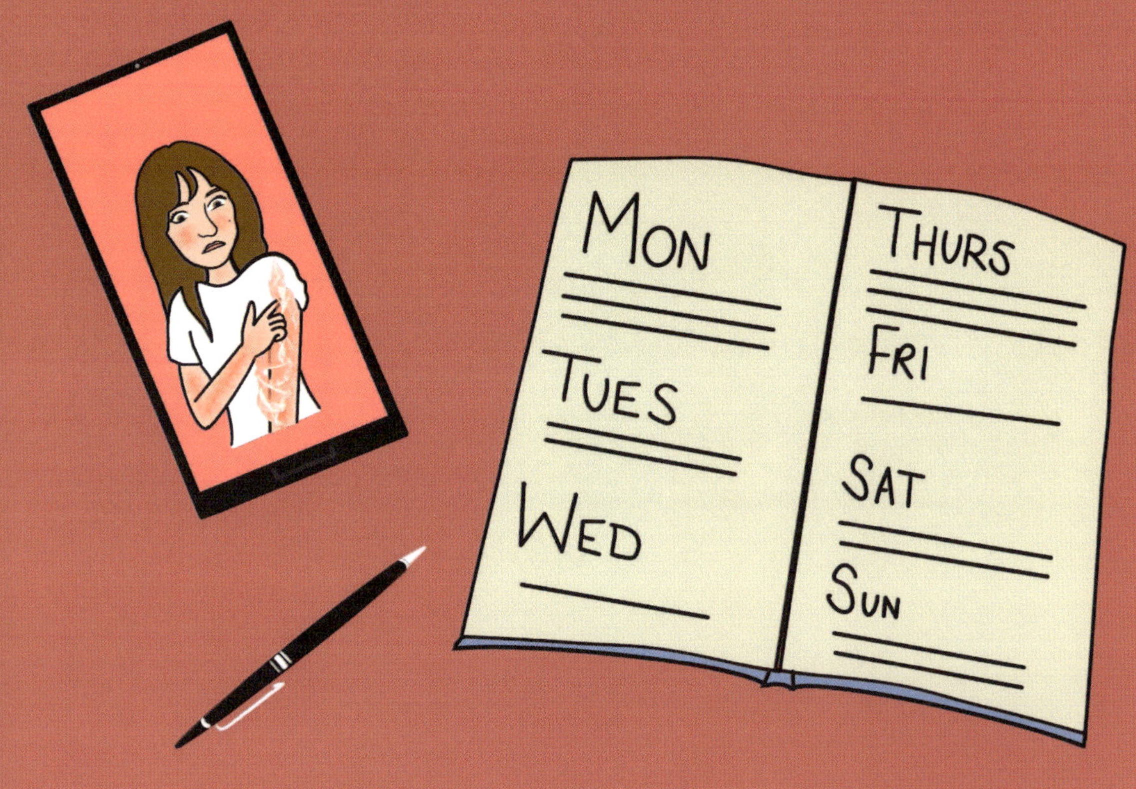
Mon
Tues
Wed
Thurs
Fri
Sat
Sun

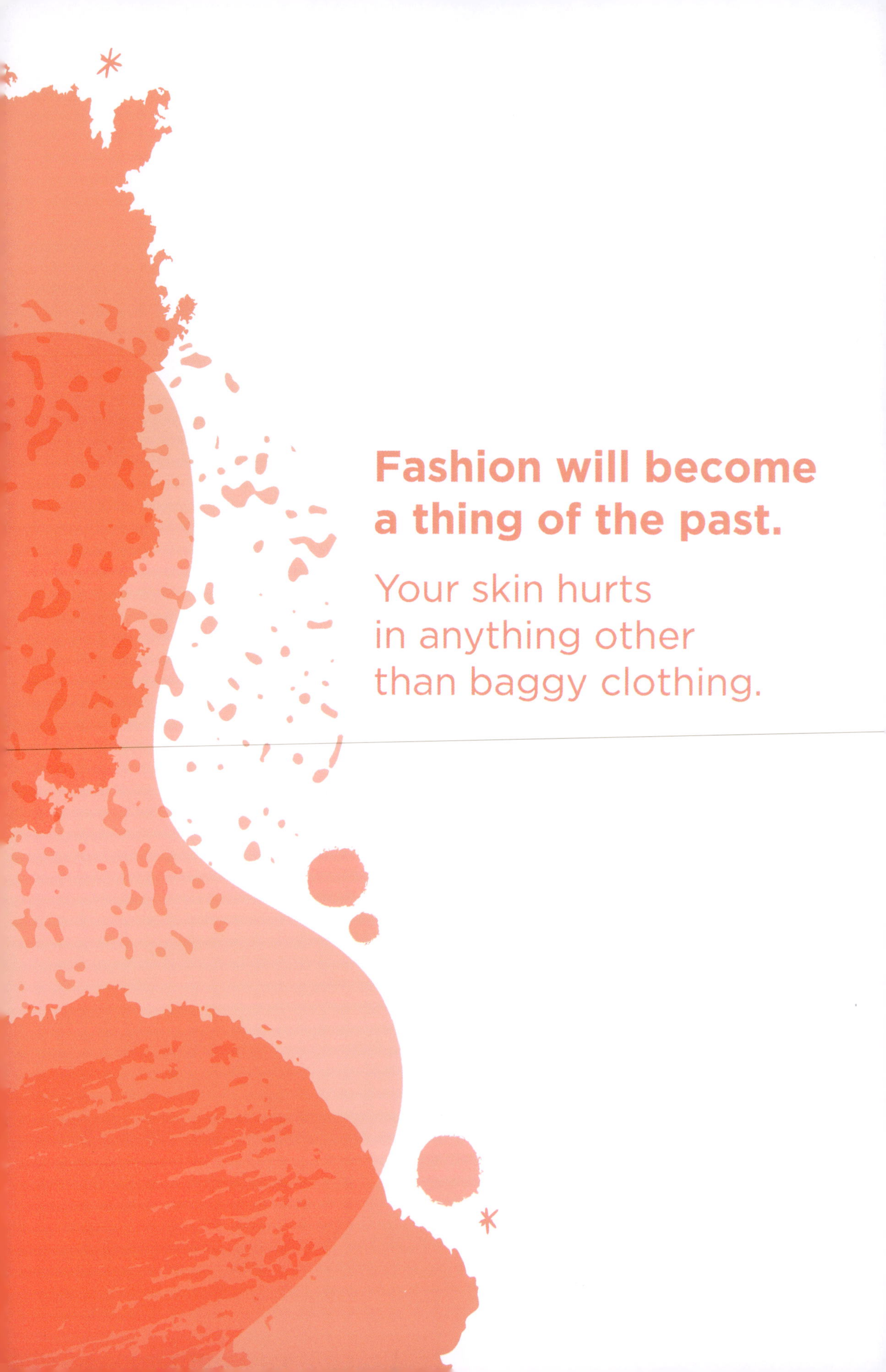

Fashion will become a thing of the past.

Your skin hurts
in anything other
than baggy clothing.

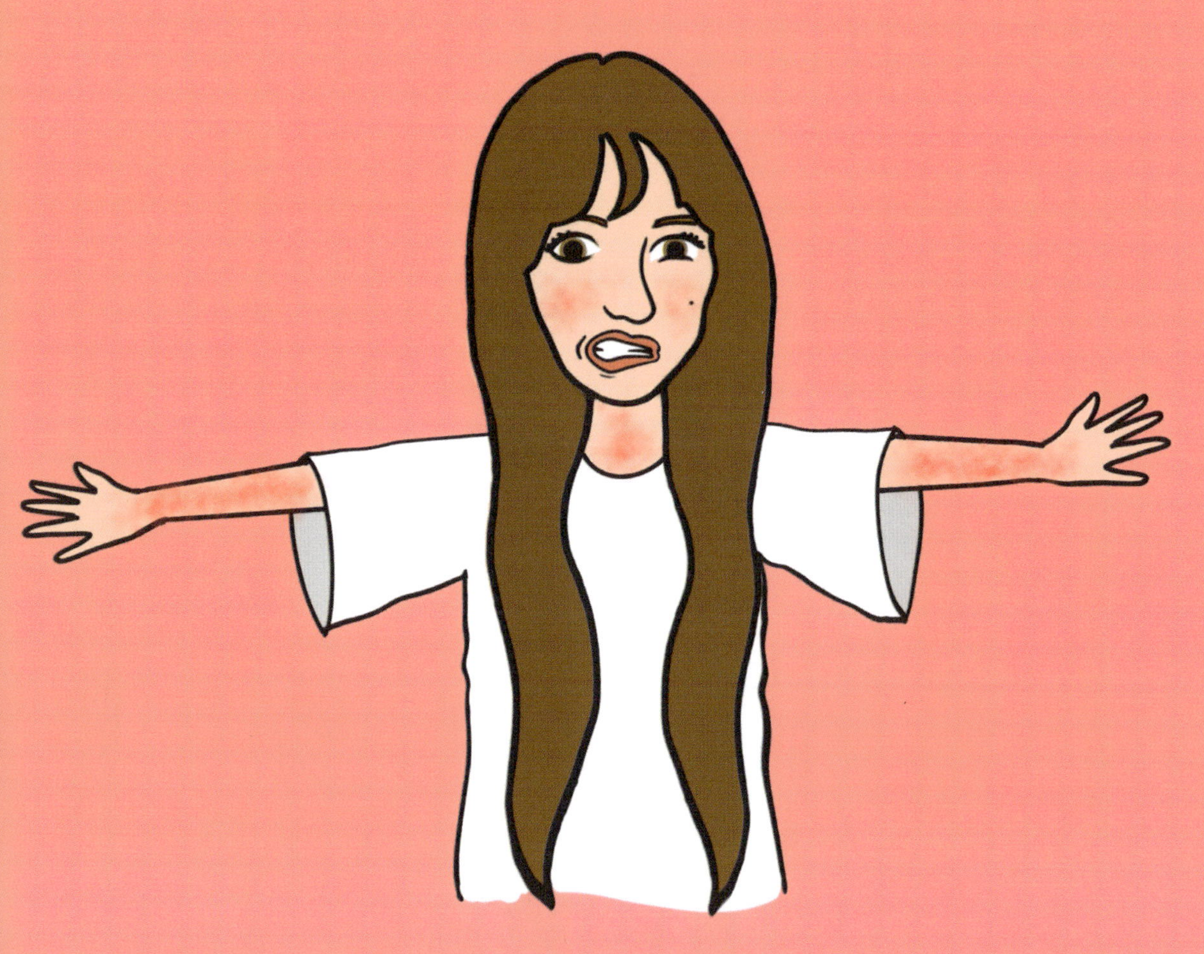

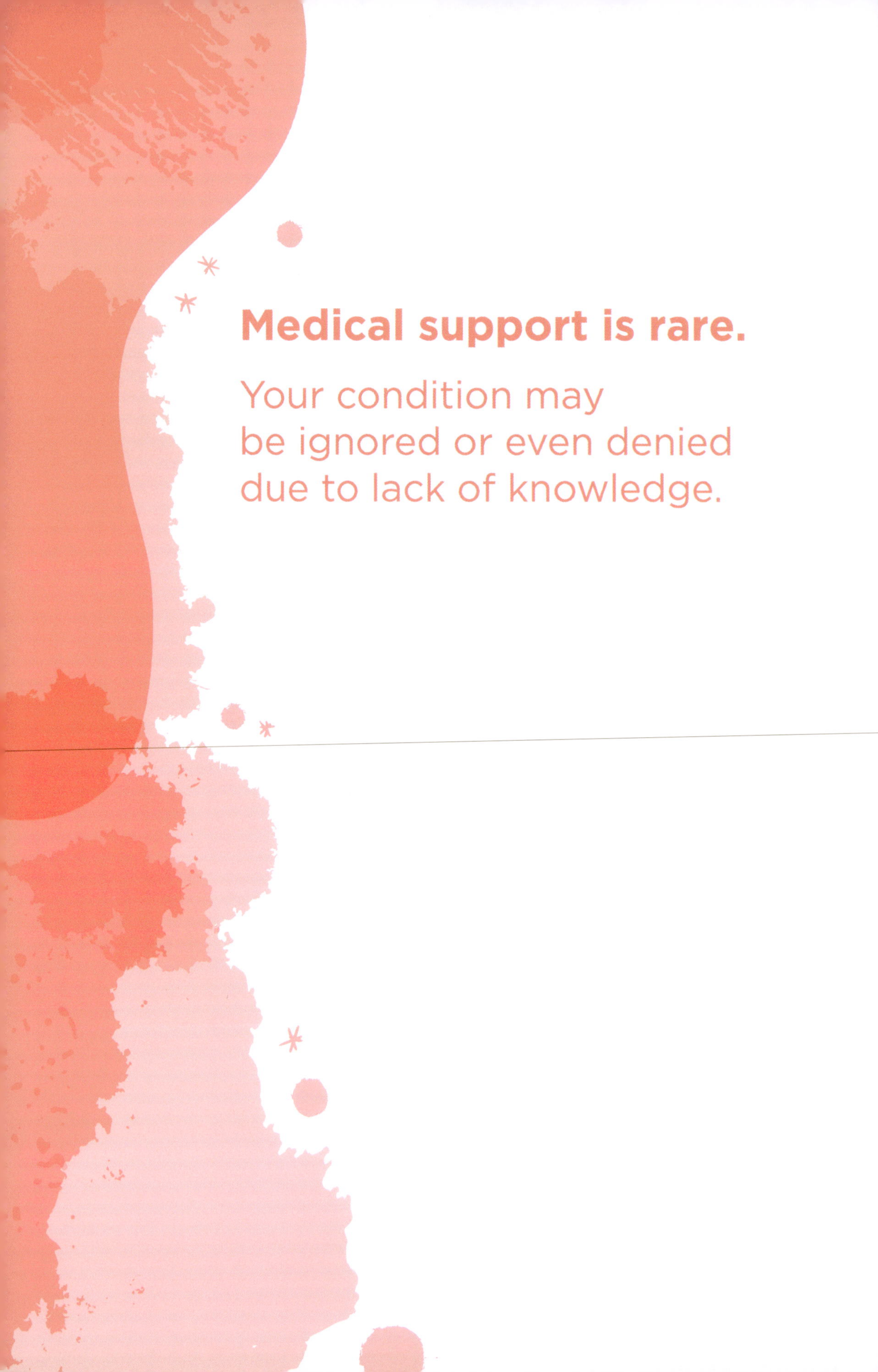

Medical support is rare.

Your condition may be ignored or even denied due to lack of knowledge.

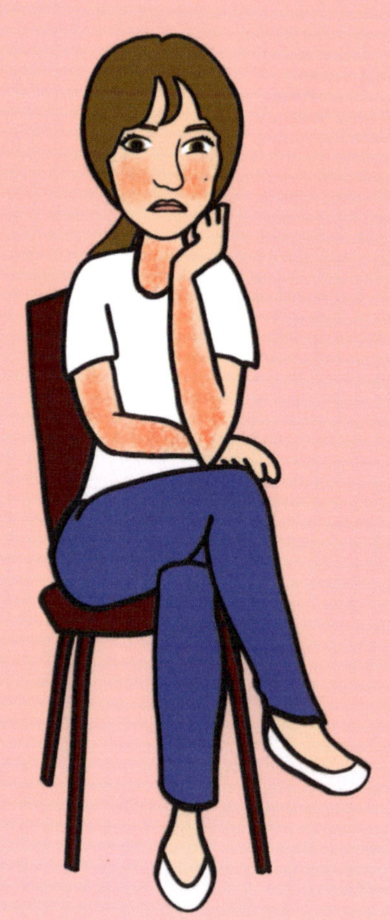

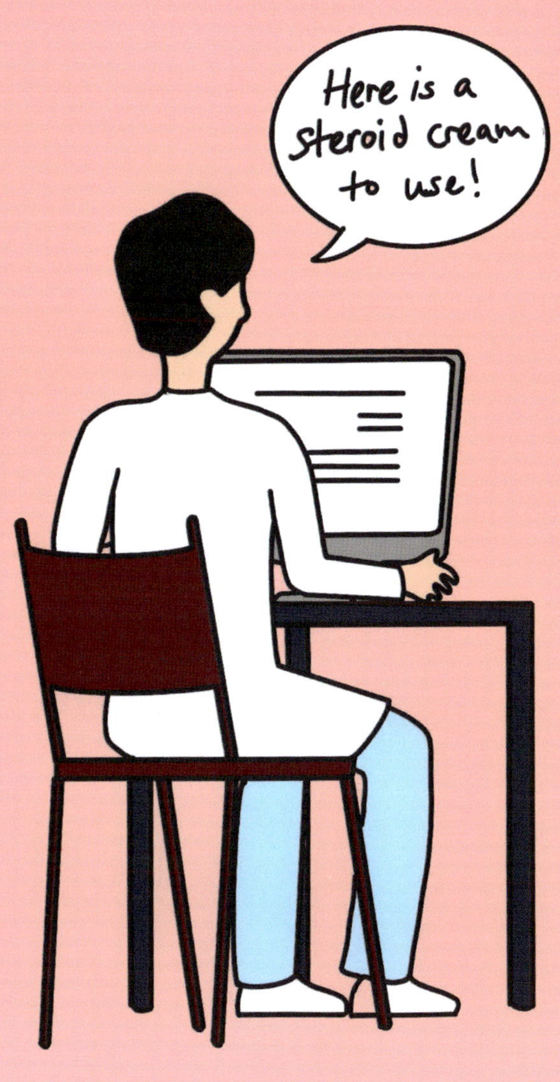

Here is a
steroid cream
to use!

It will be an emotional ride.

You'll feel angry about all of this.
That's OK.

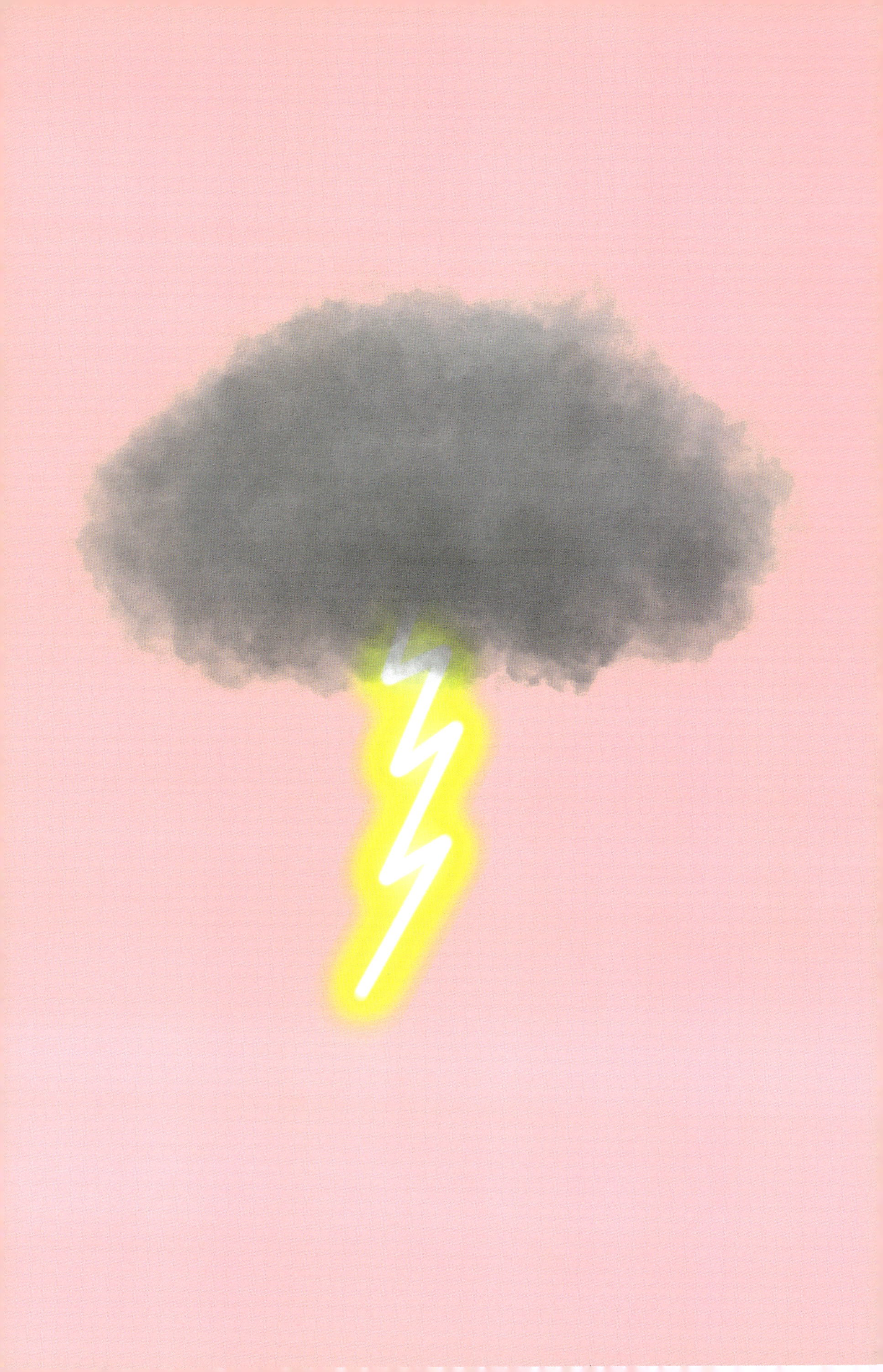

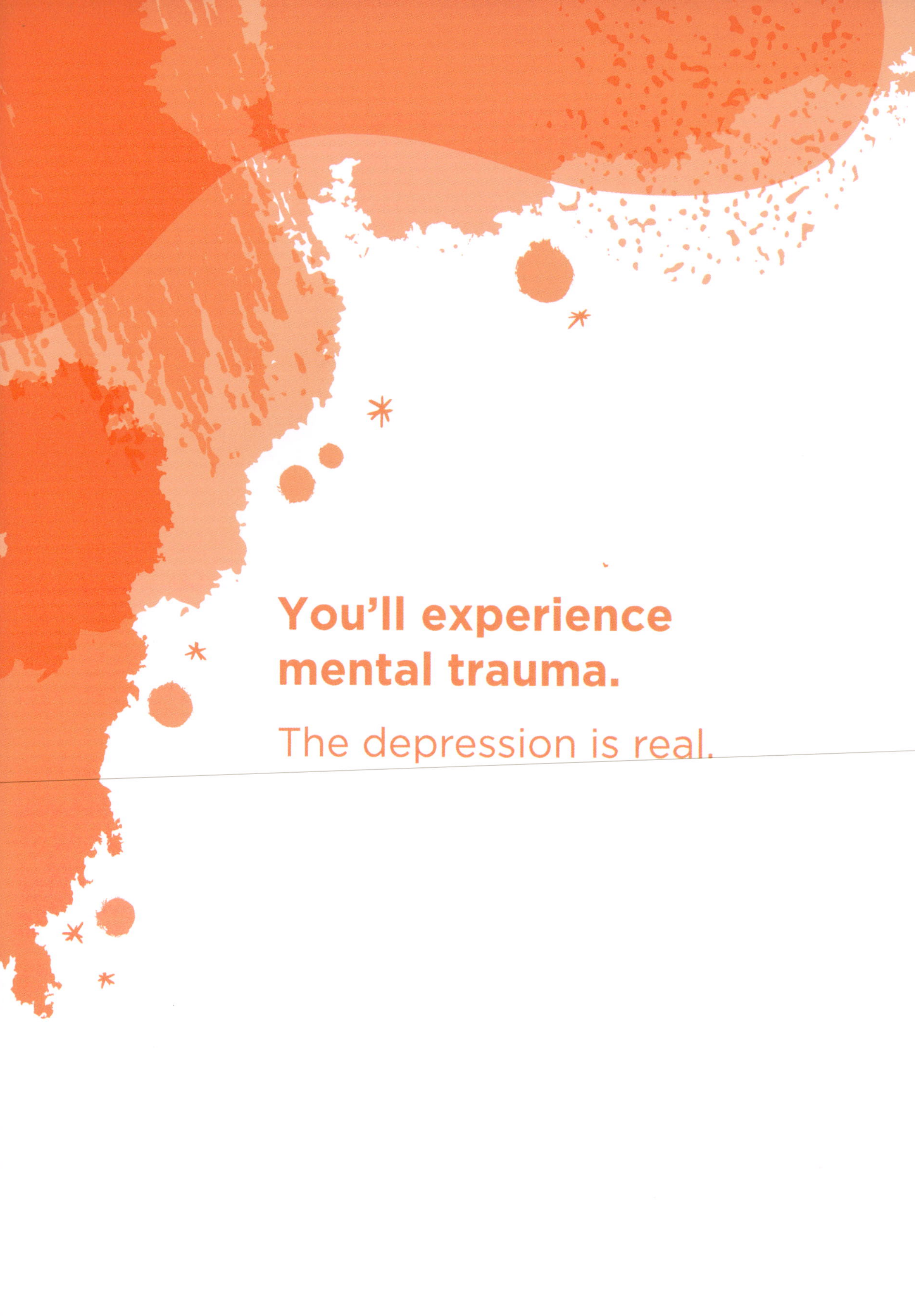

You'll experience mental trauma.

The depression is real.

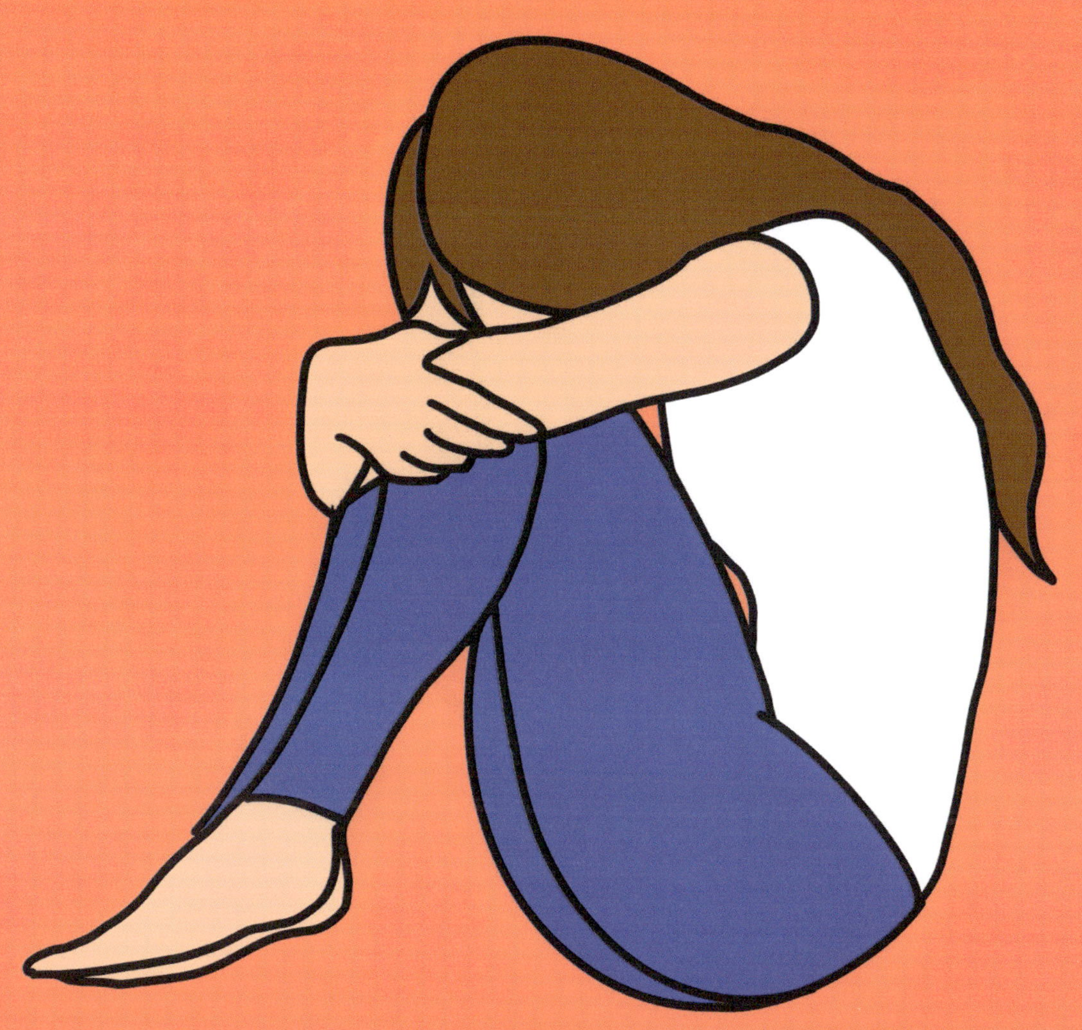

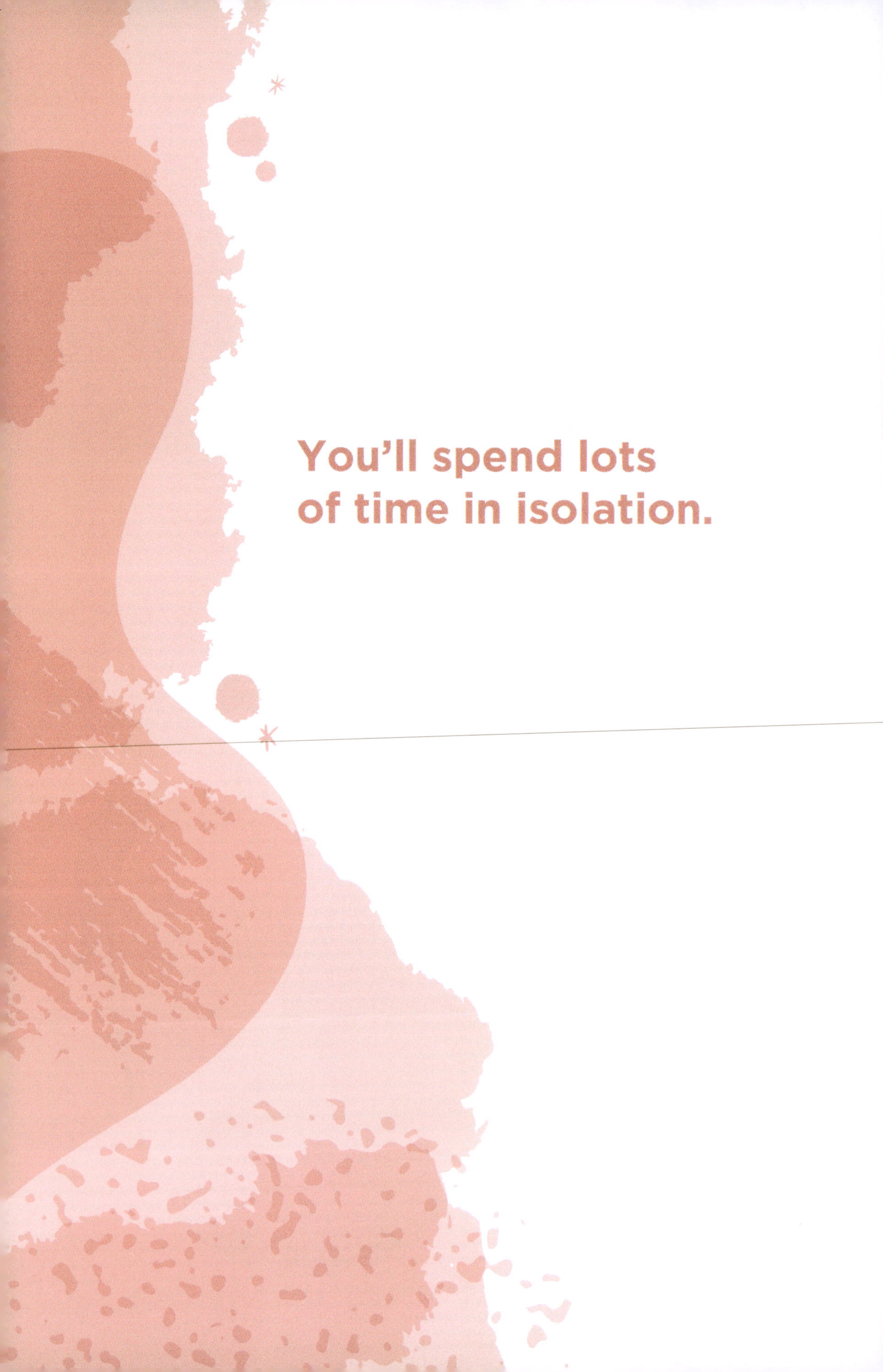

You'll spend lots
of time in isolation.

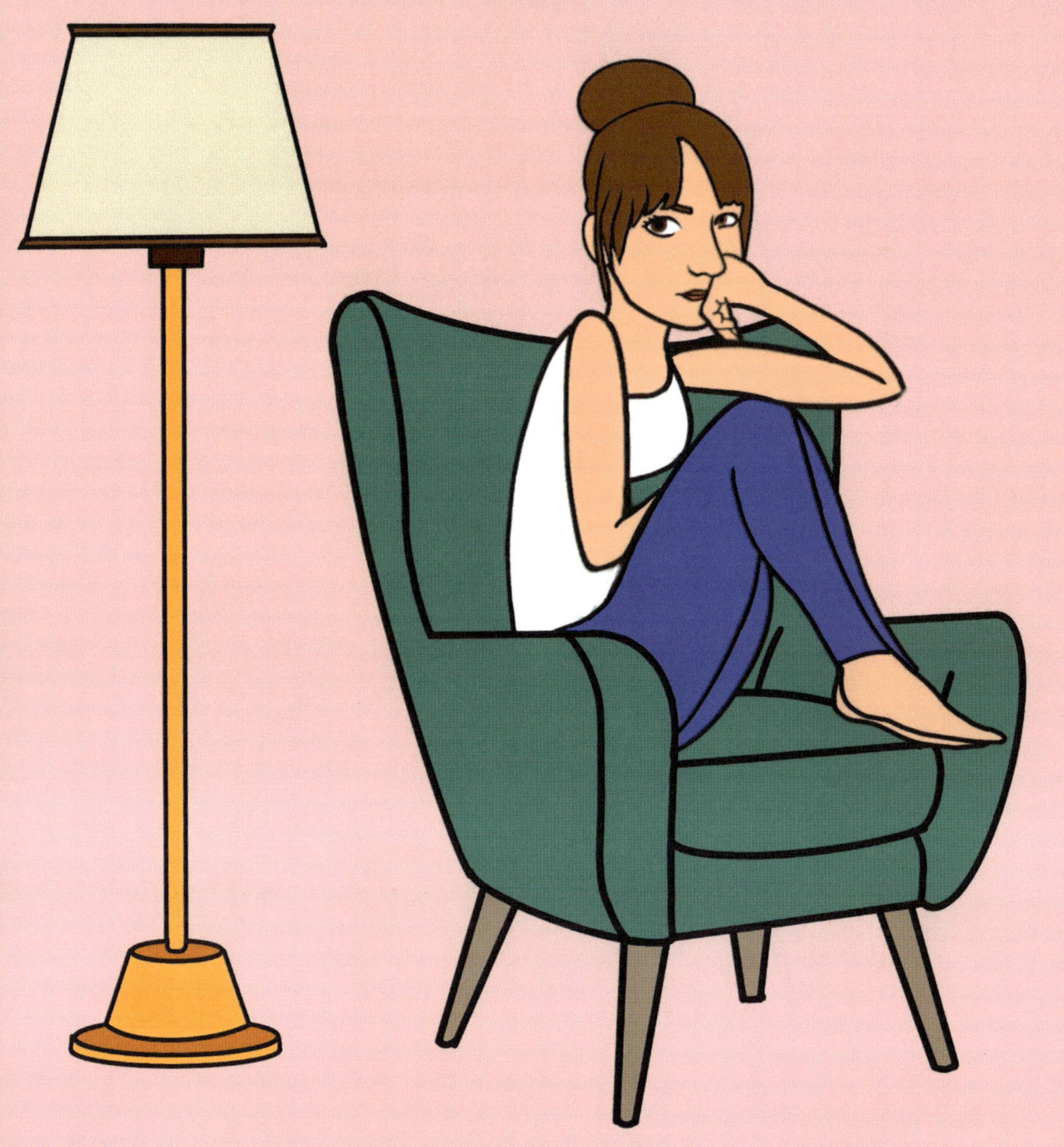

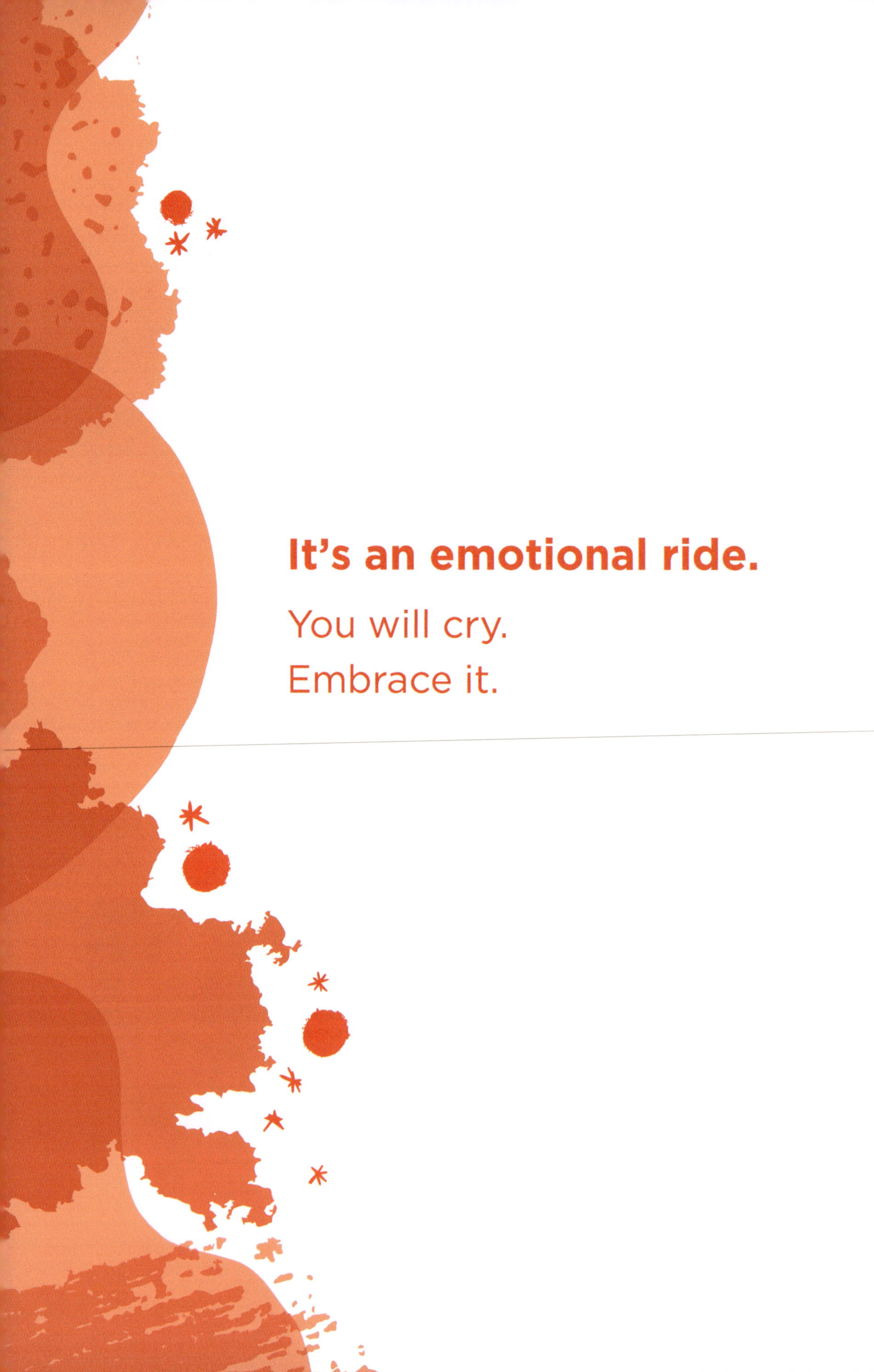

It's an emotional ride.

You will cry.

Embrace it.

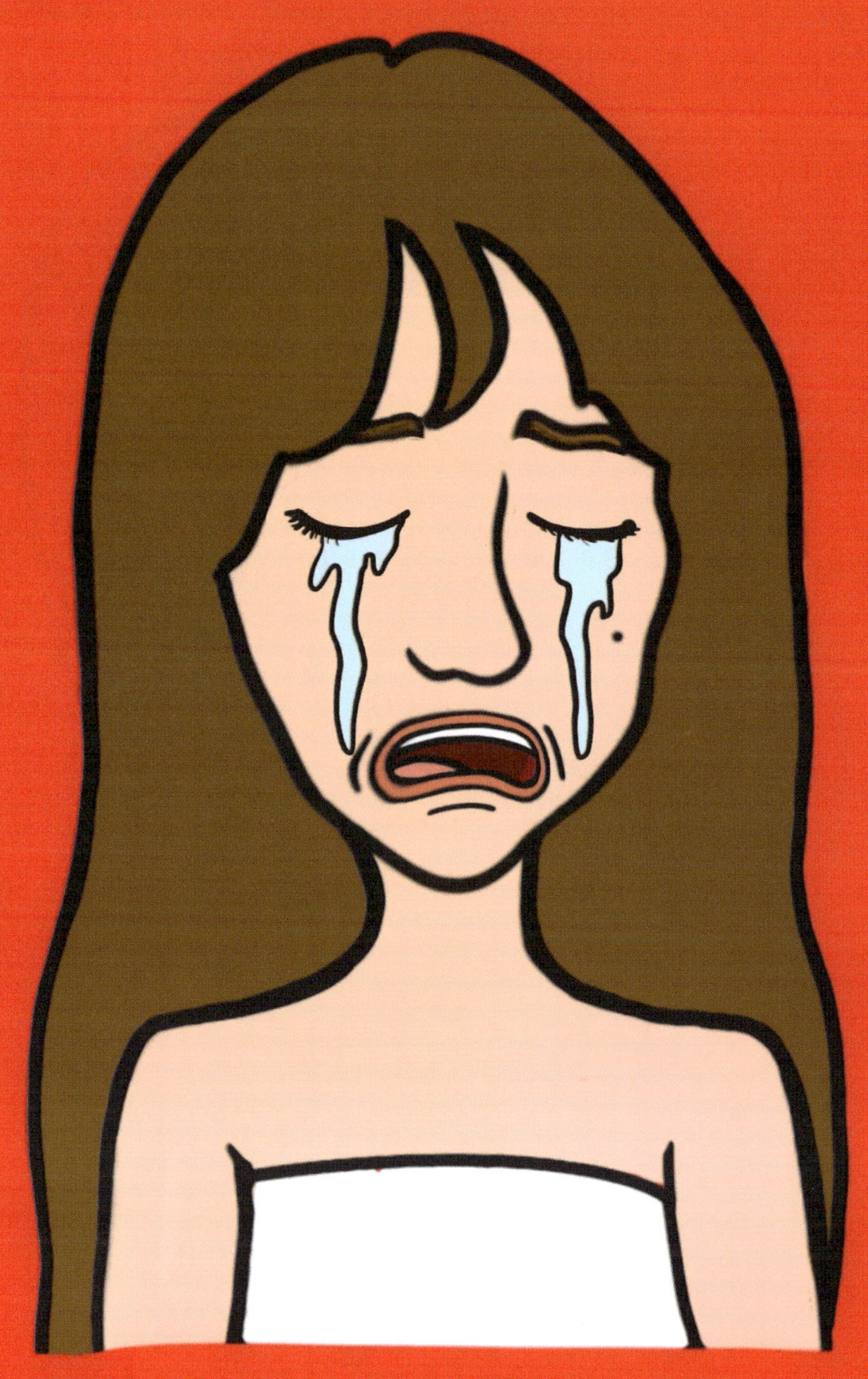

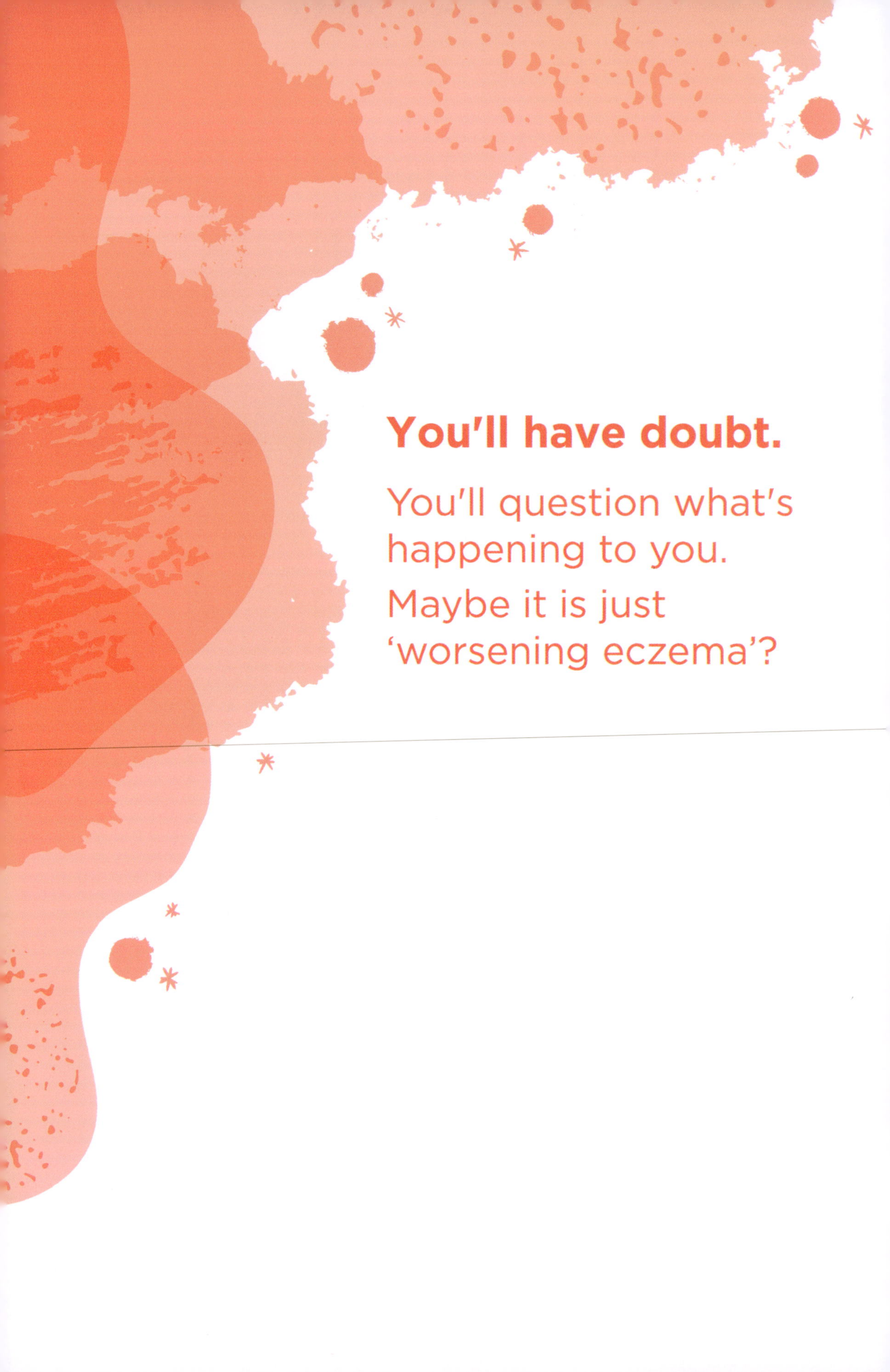

You'll have doubt.

You'll question what's happening to you.

Maybe it is just 'worsening eczema'?

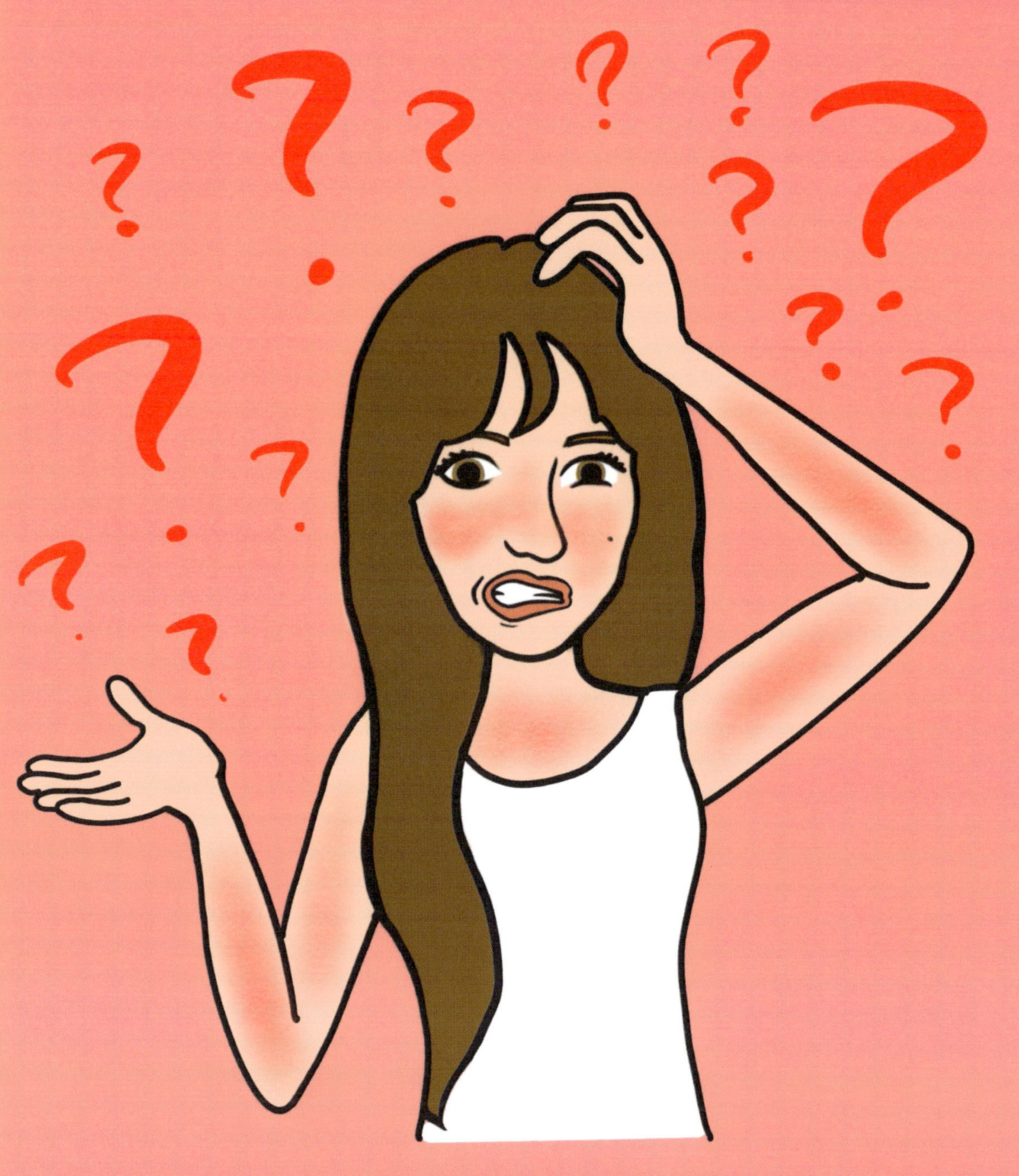

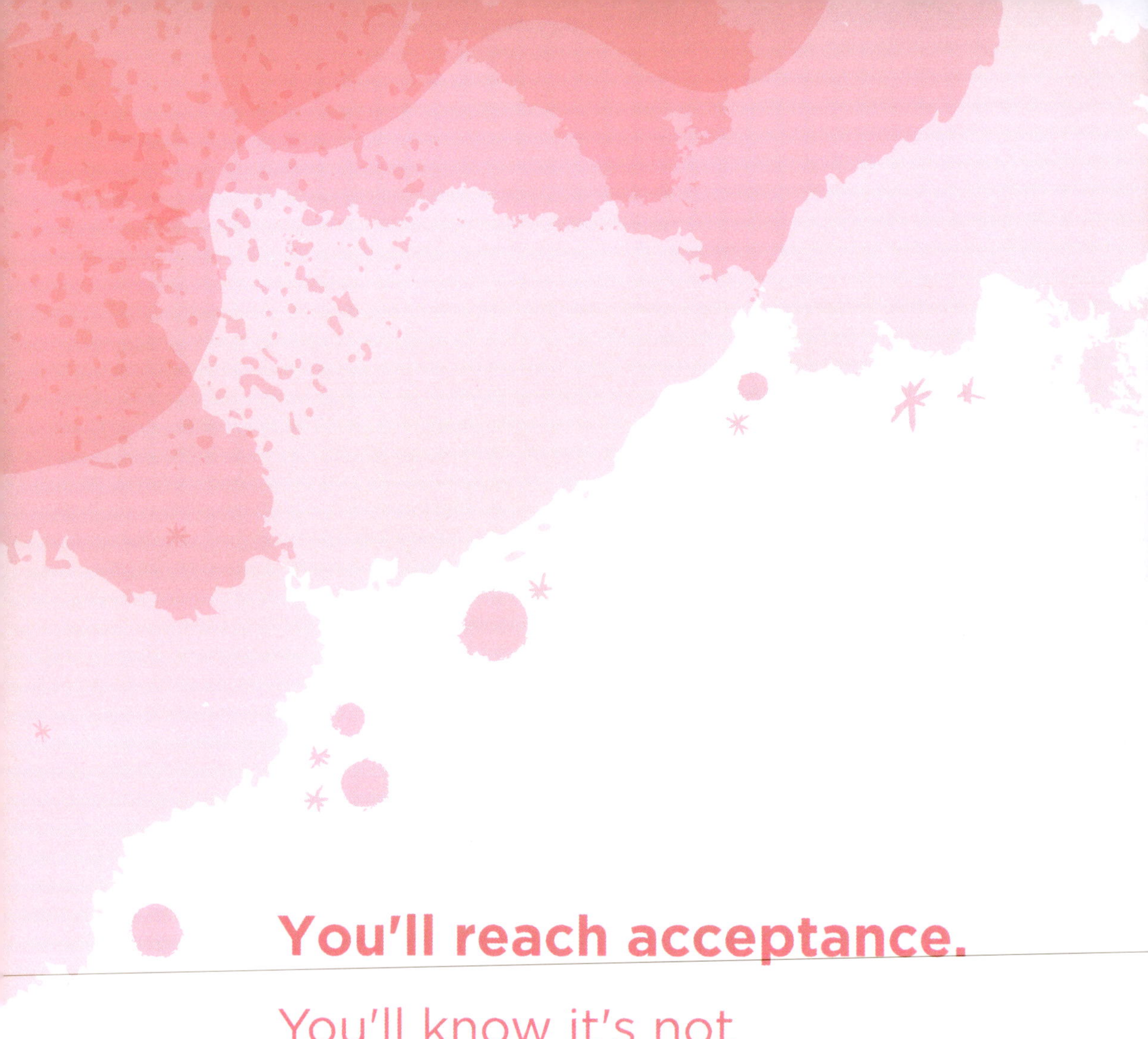

You'll reach acceptance.

You'll know it's not 'worsening eczema'.

You'll know your body is recovering from the eczema medication.

You'll accept you have TSW and KNOW you'll heal.

You'll accept what it is and begin to heal.

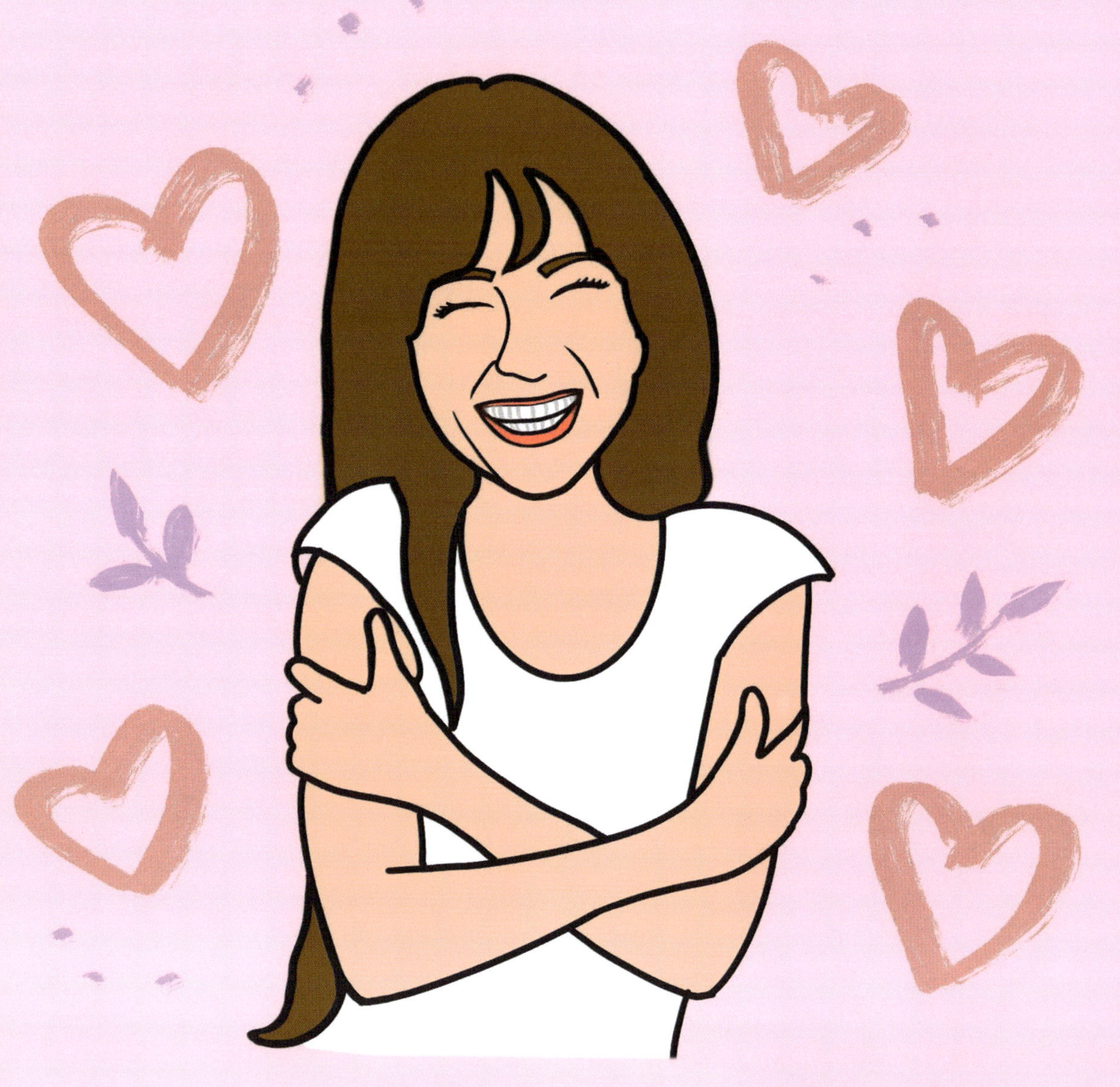

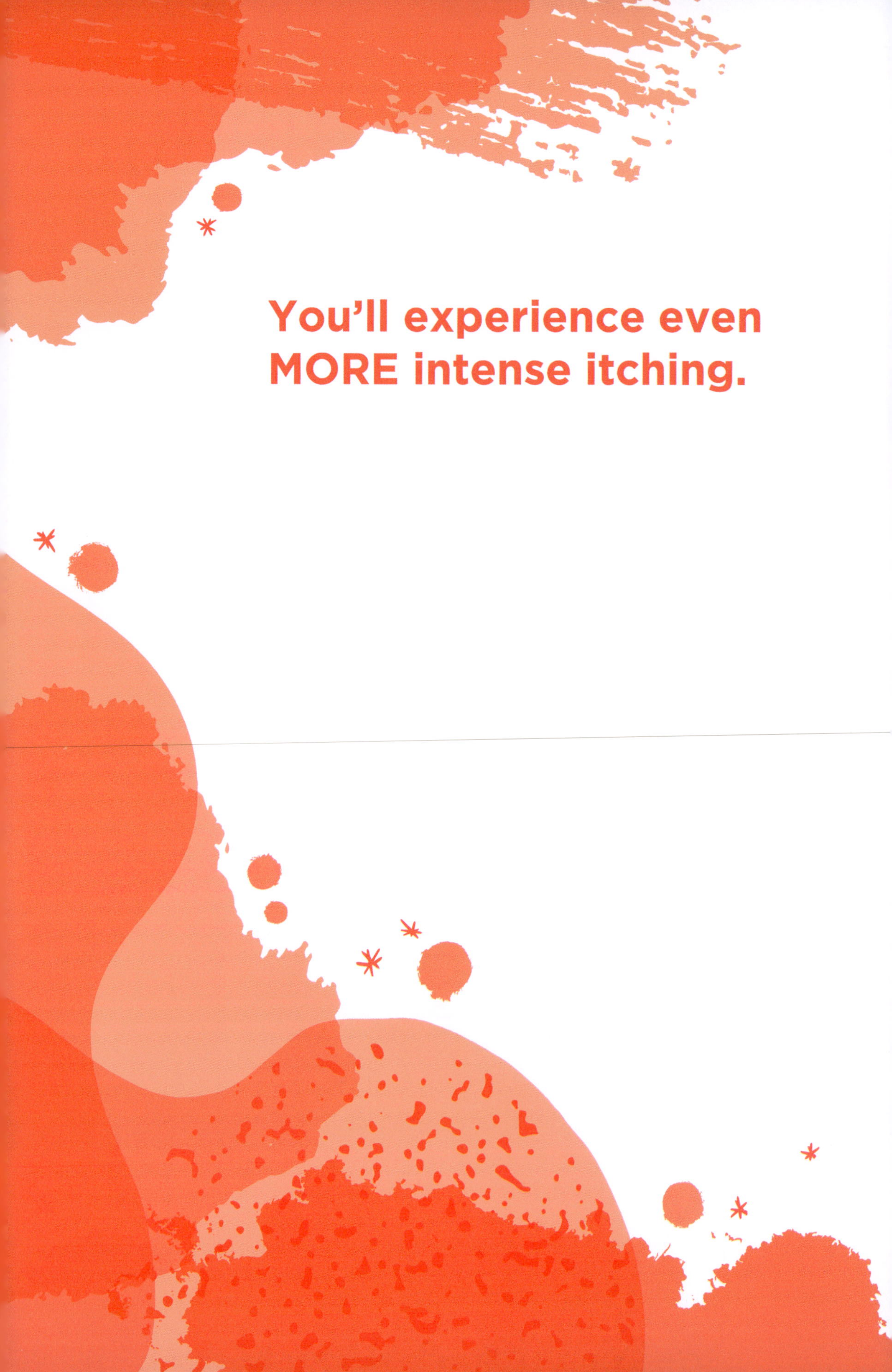

You'll experience even MORE intense itching.

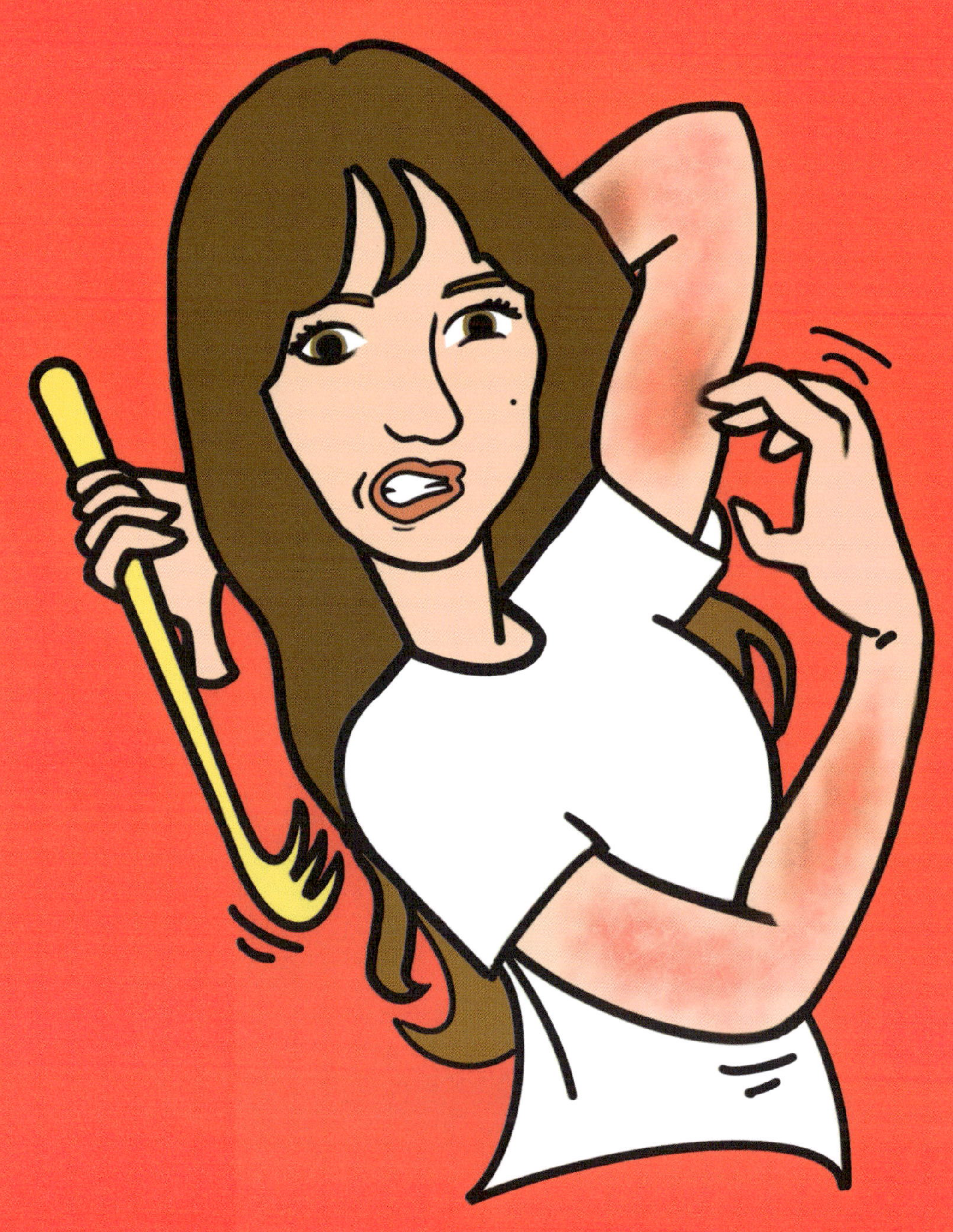

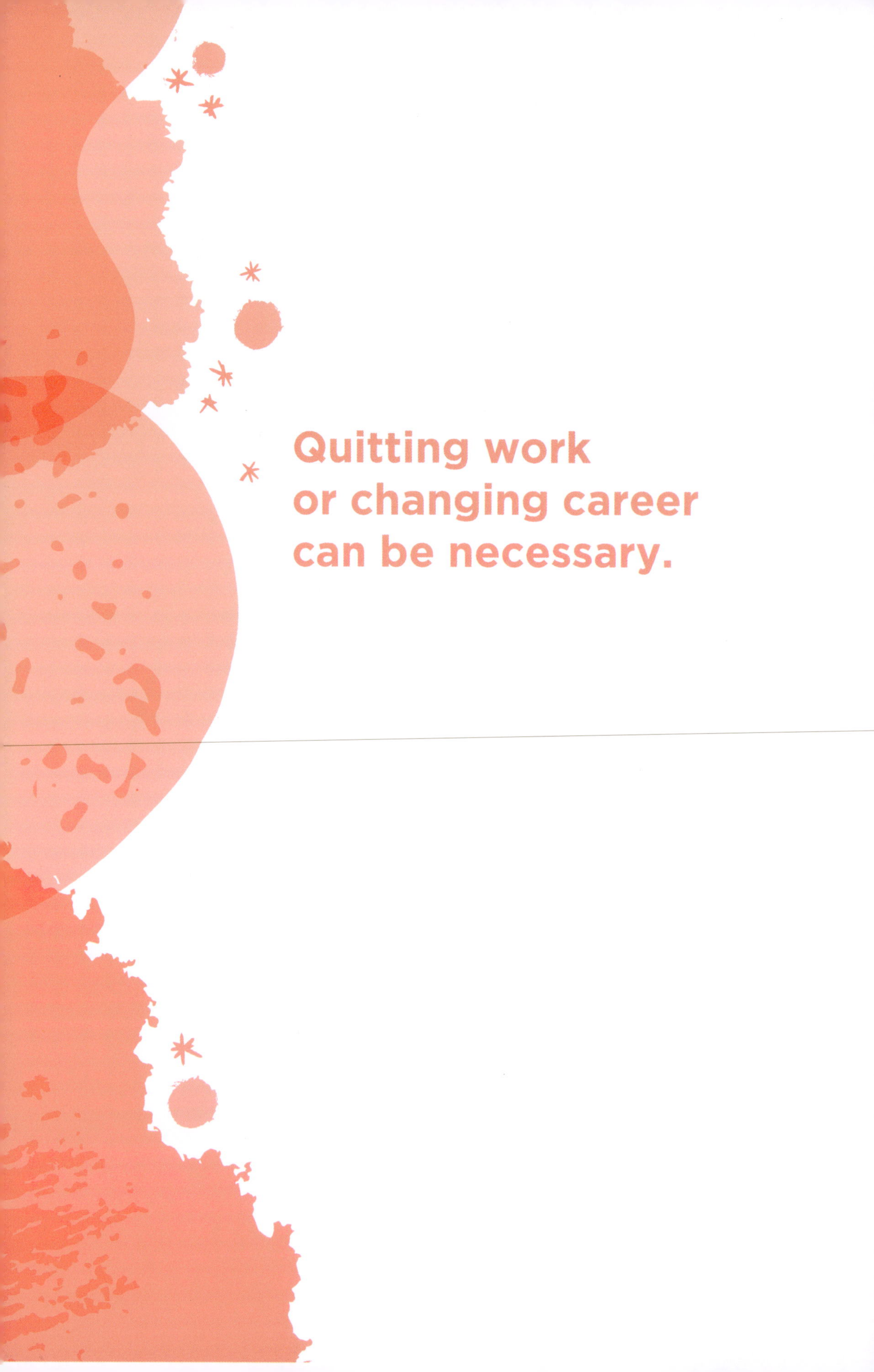

Quitting work
or changing career
can be necessary.

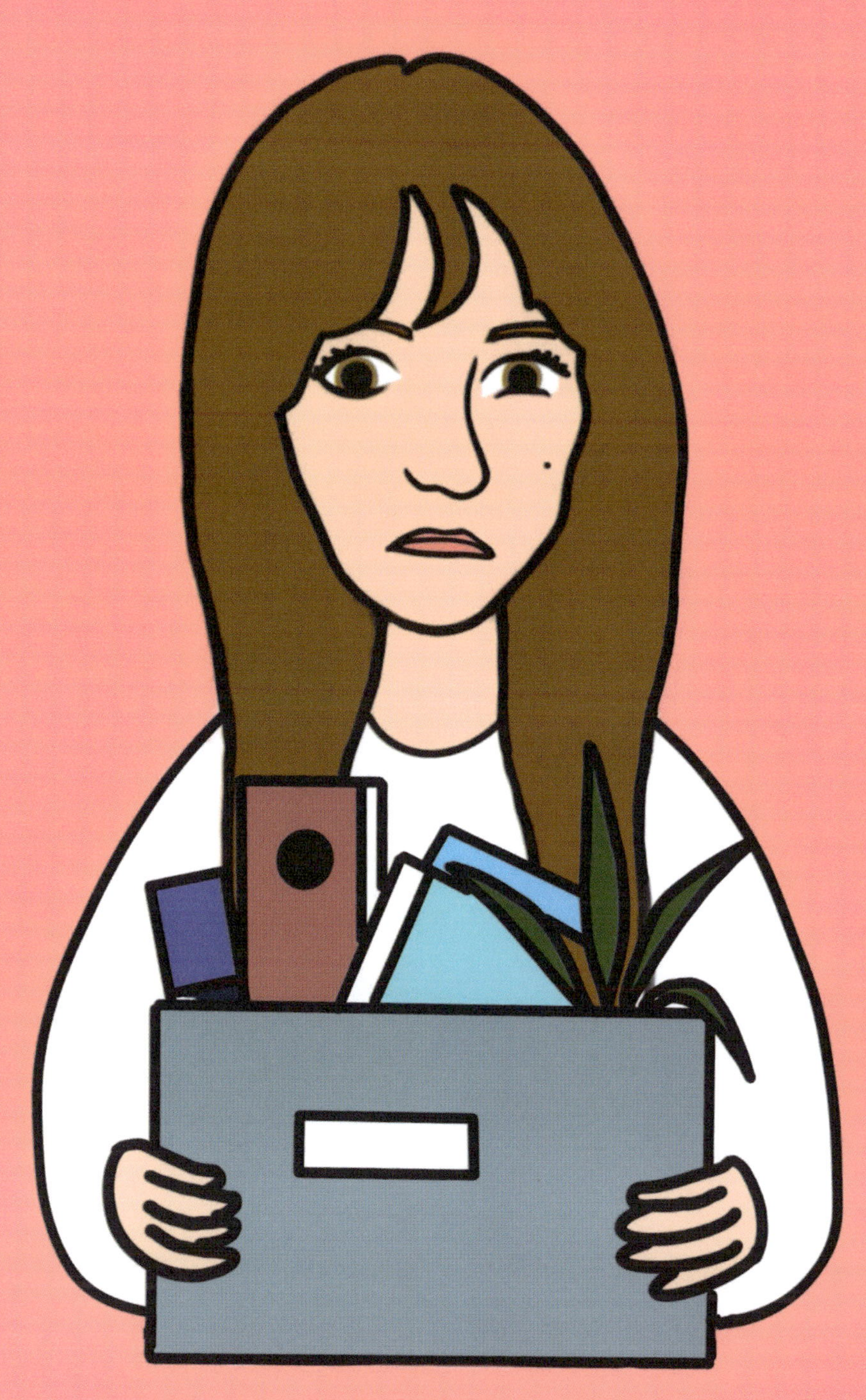

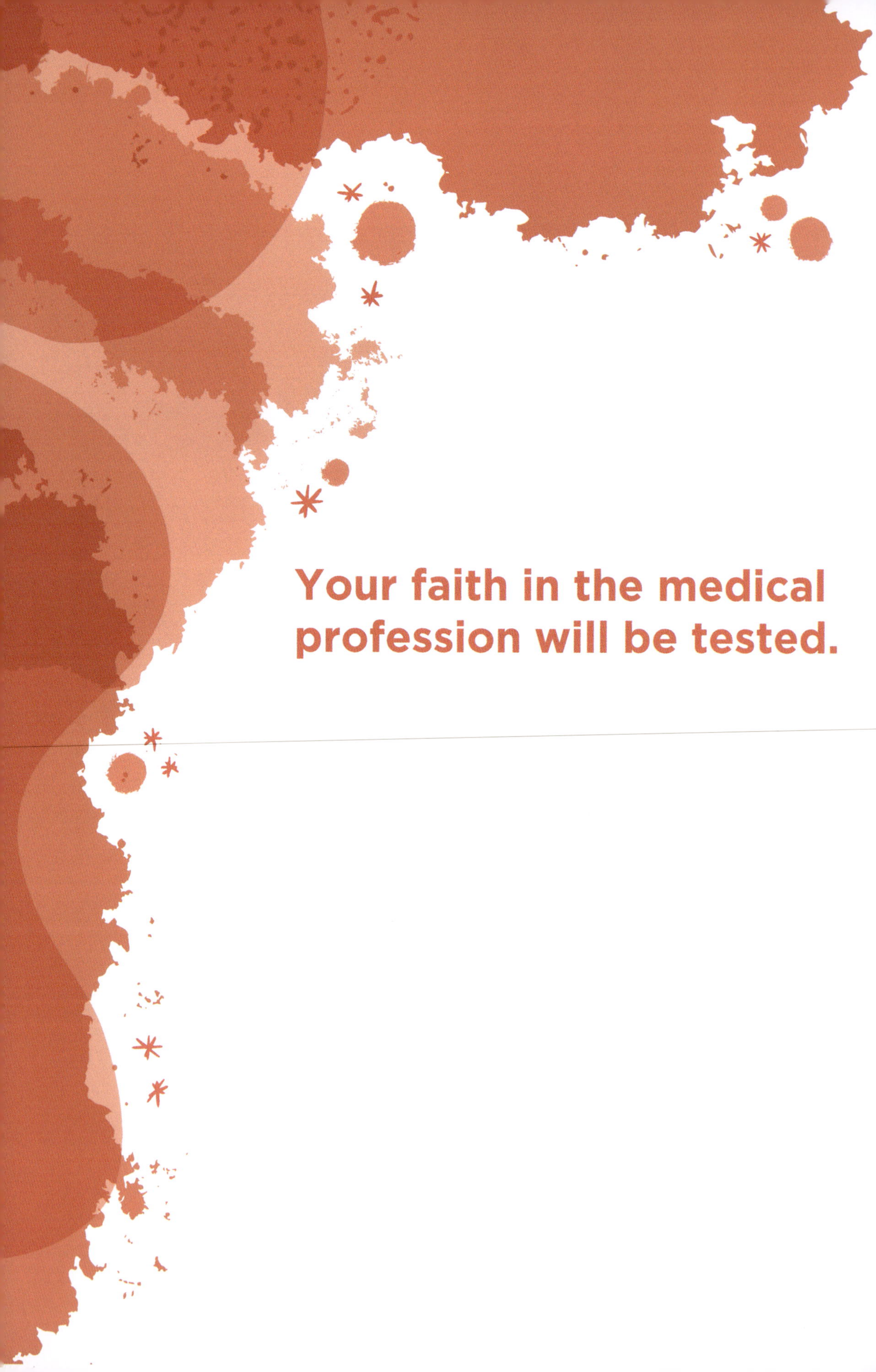
Your faith in the medical
profession will be tested.

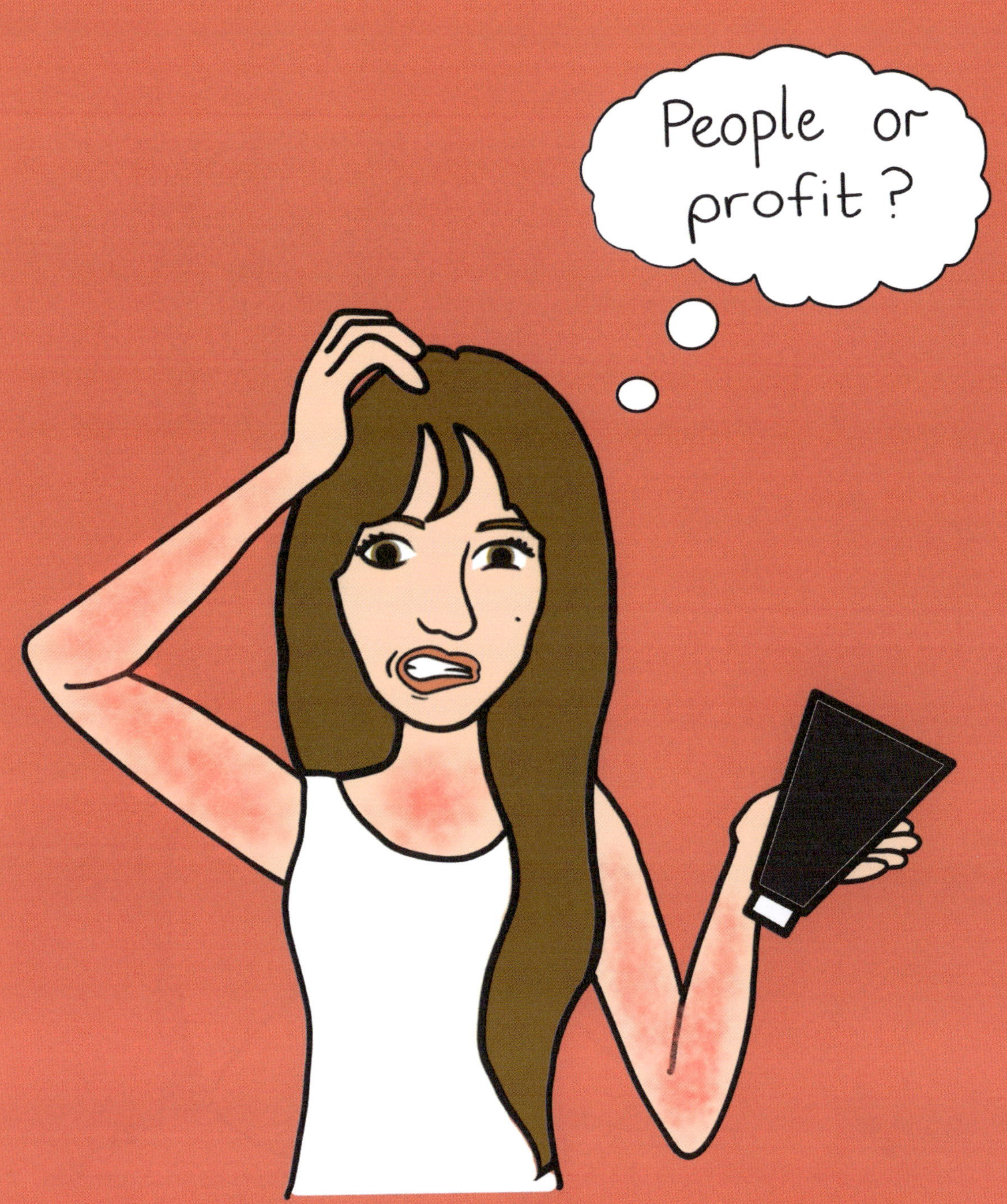
People or profit?

You'd do anything
for an end date.

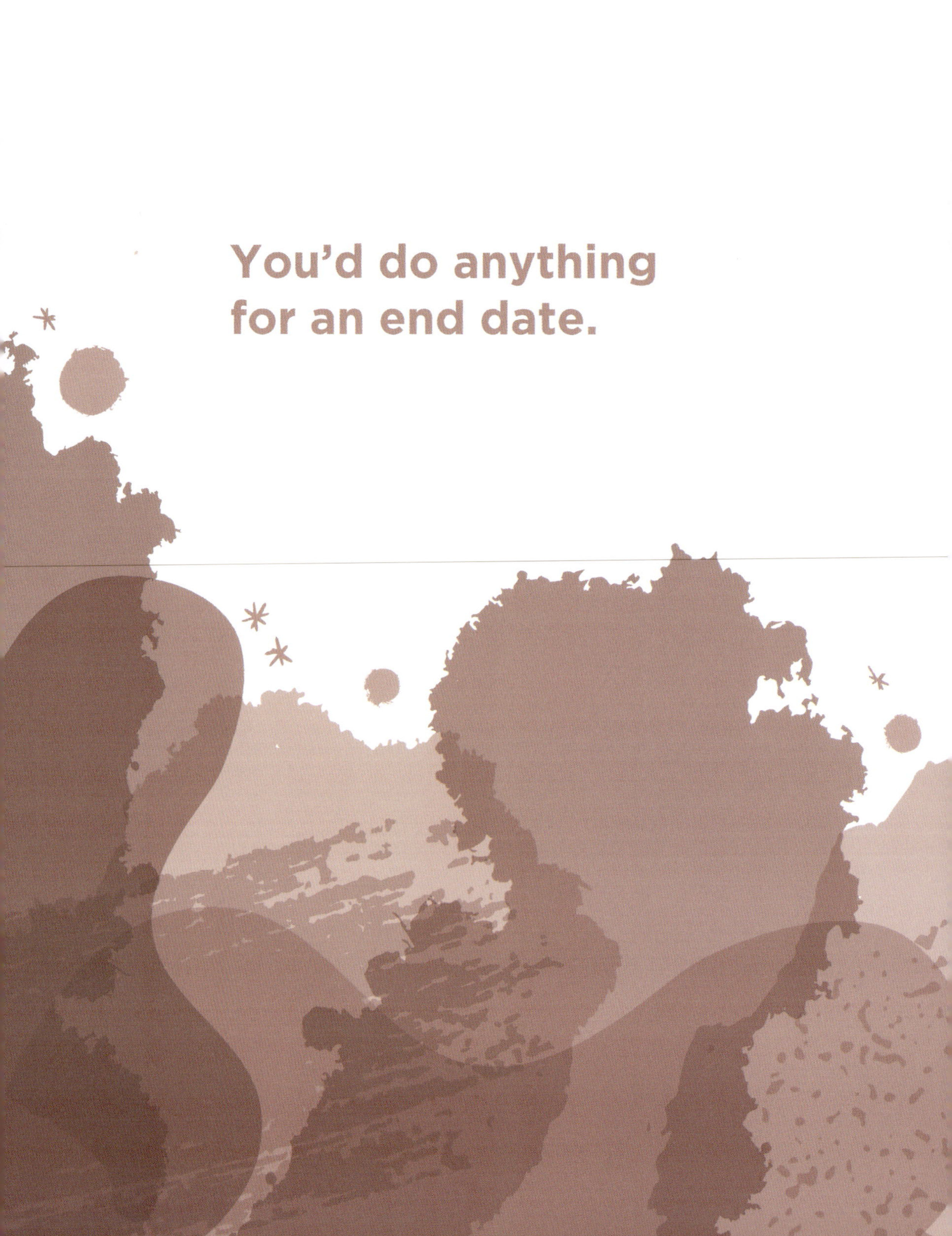

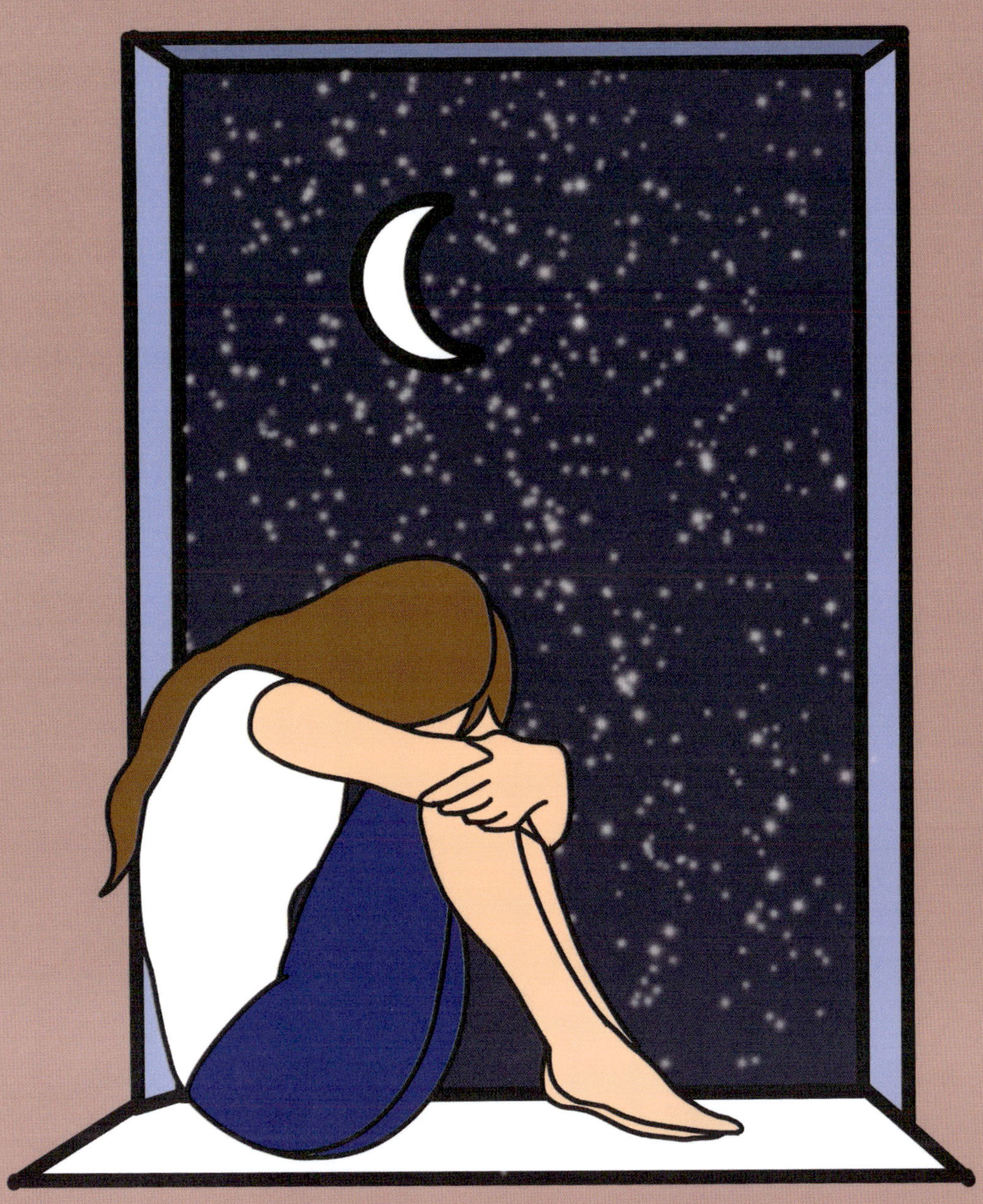

Exercise hurts.

But you know you have to do it to heal. You'll be determined.

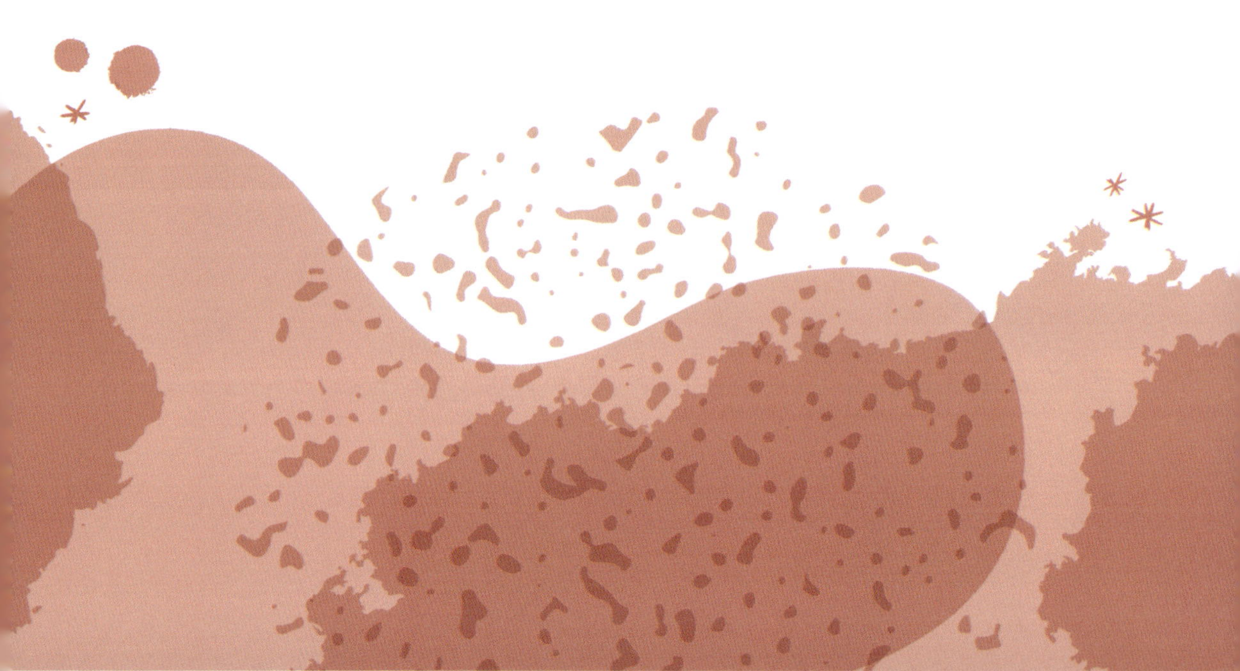

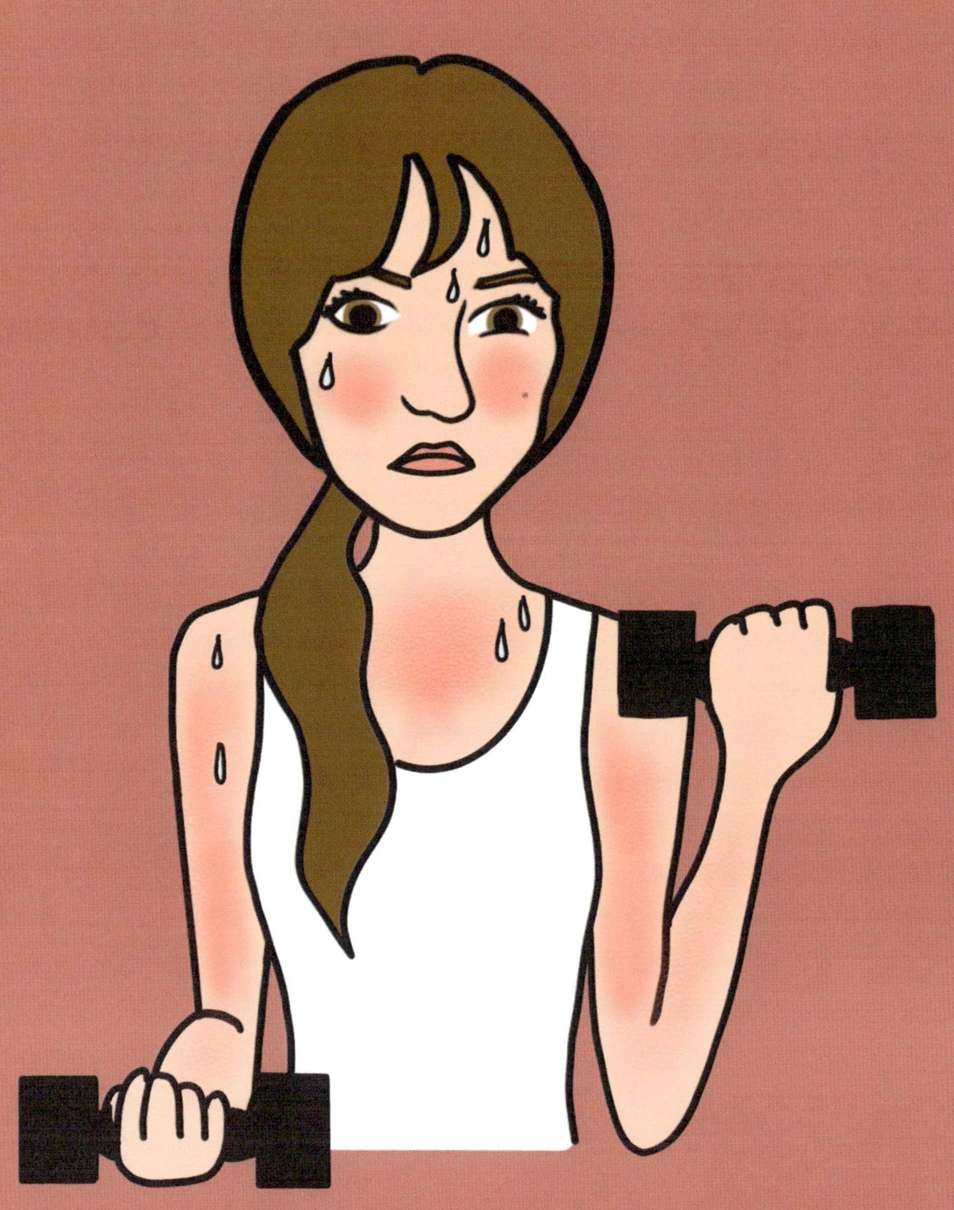

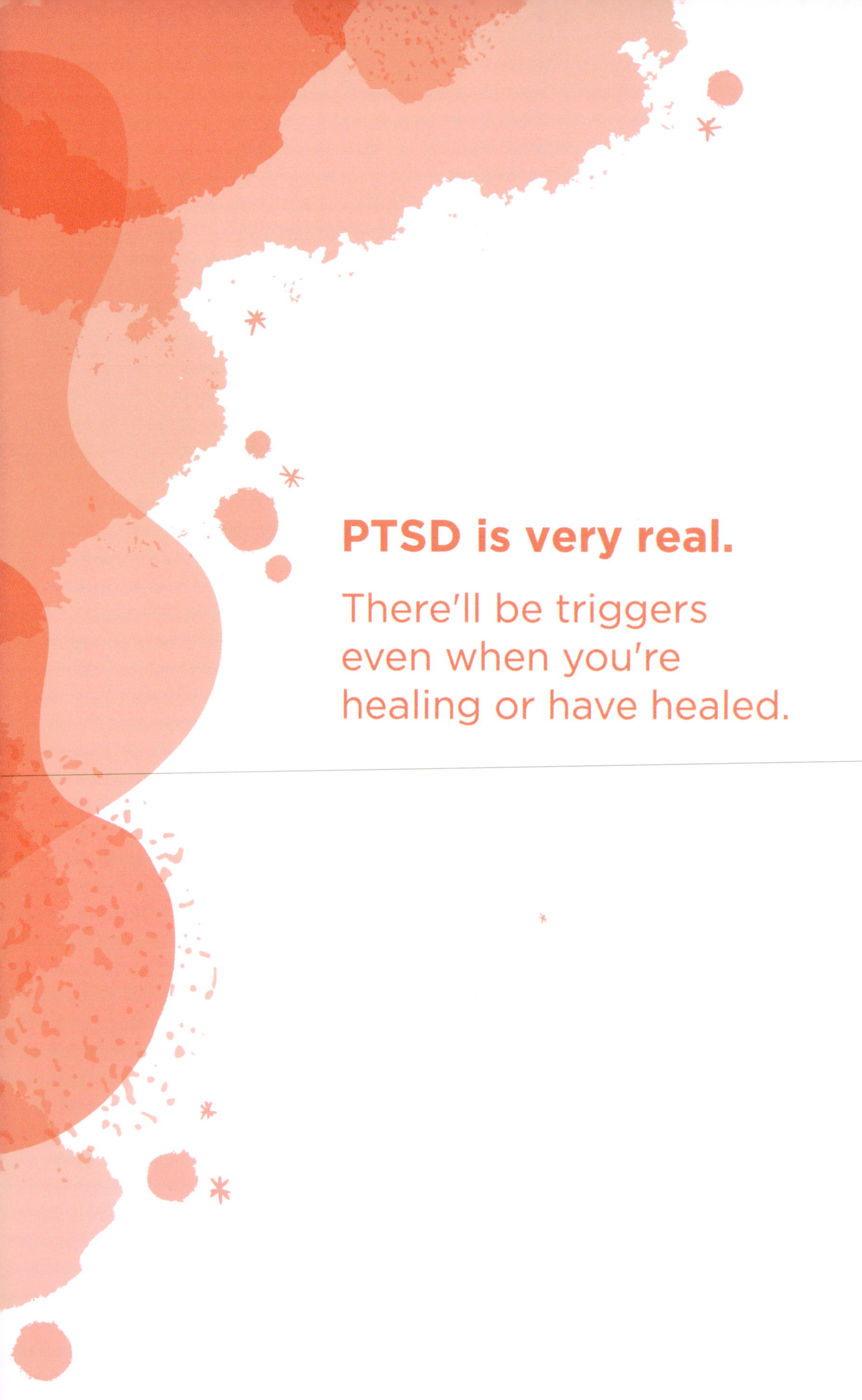

PTSD is very real.

There'll be triggers even when you're healing or have healed.

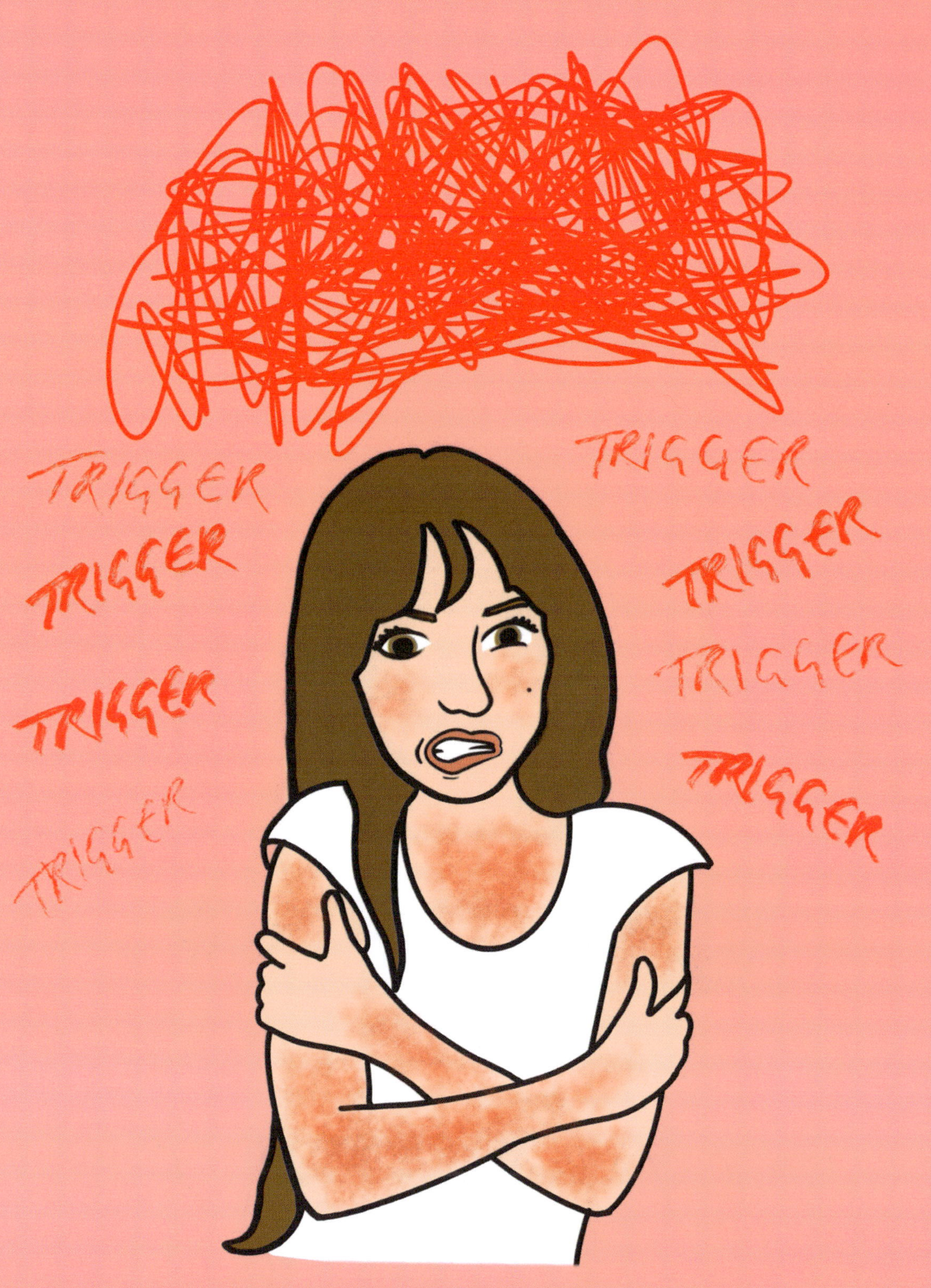
TRIGGER
TRIGGER
TRIGGER
TRIGGER
TRIGGER
TRIGGER
TRIGGER
TRIGGER

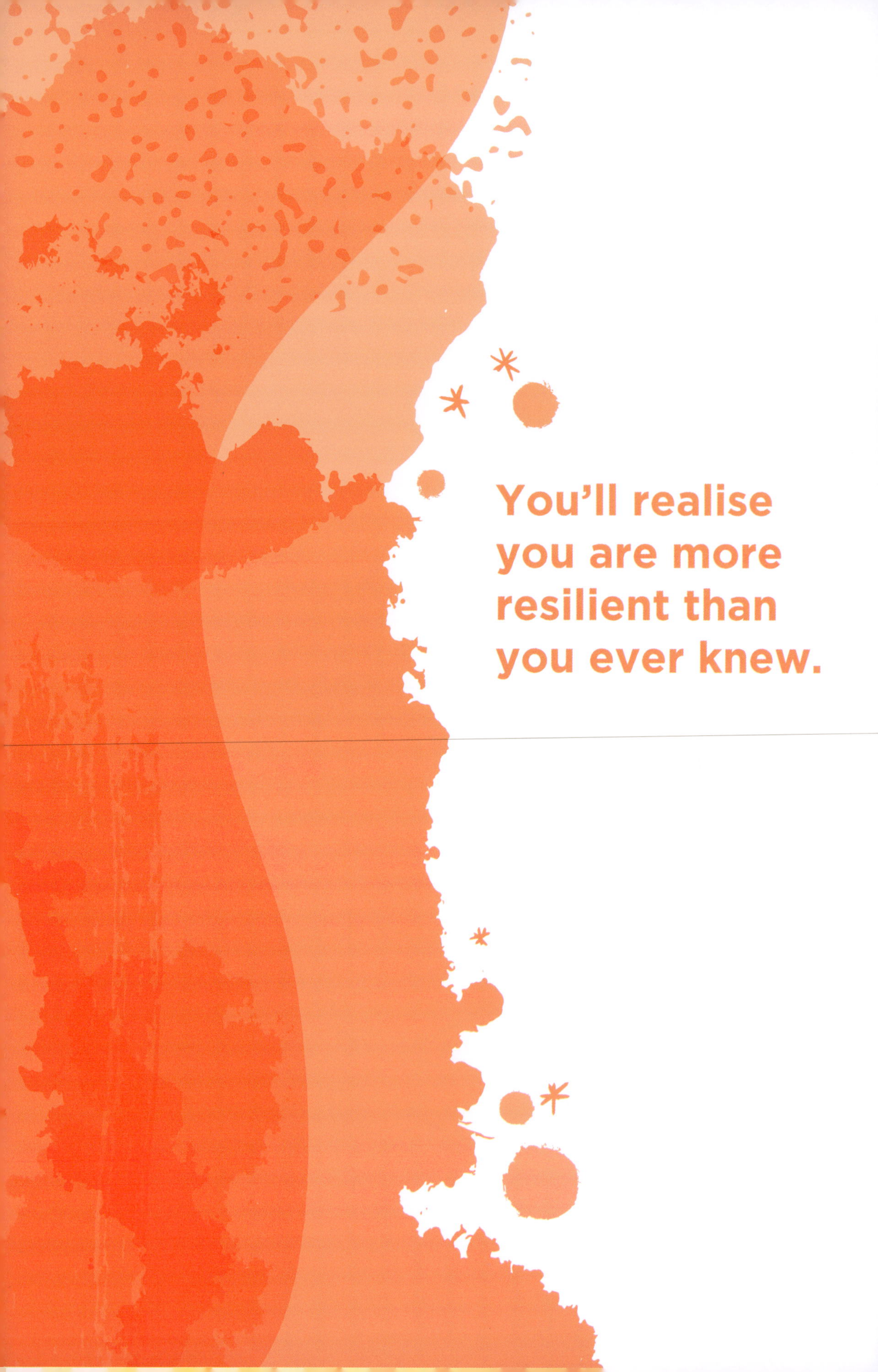
You'll realise
you are more
resilient than
you ever knew.

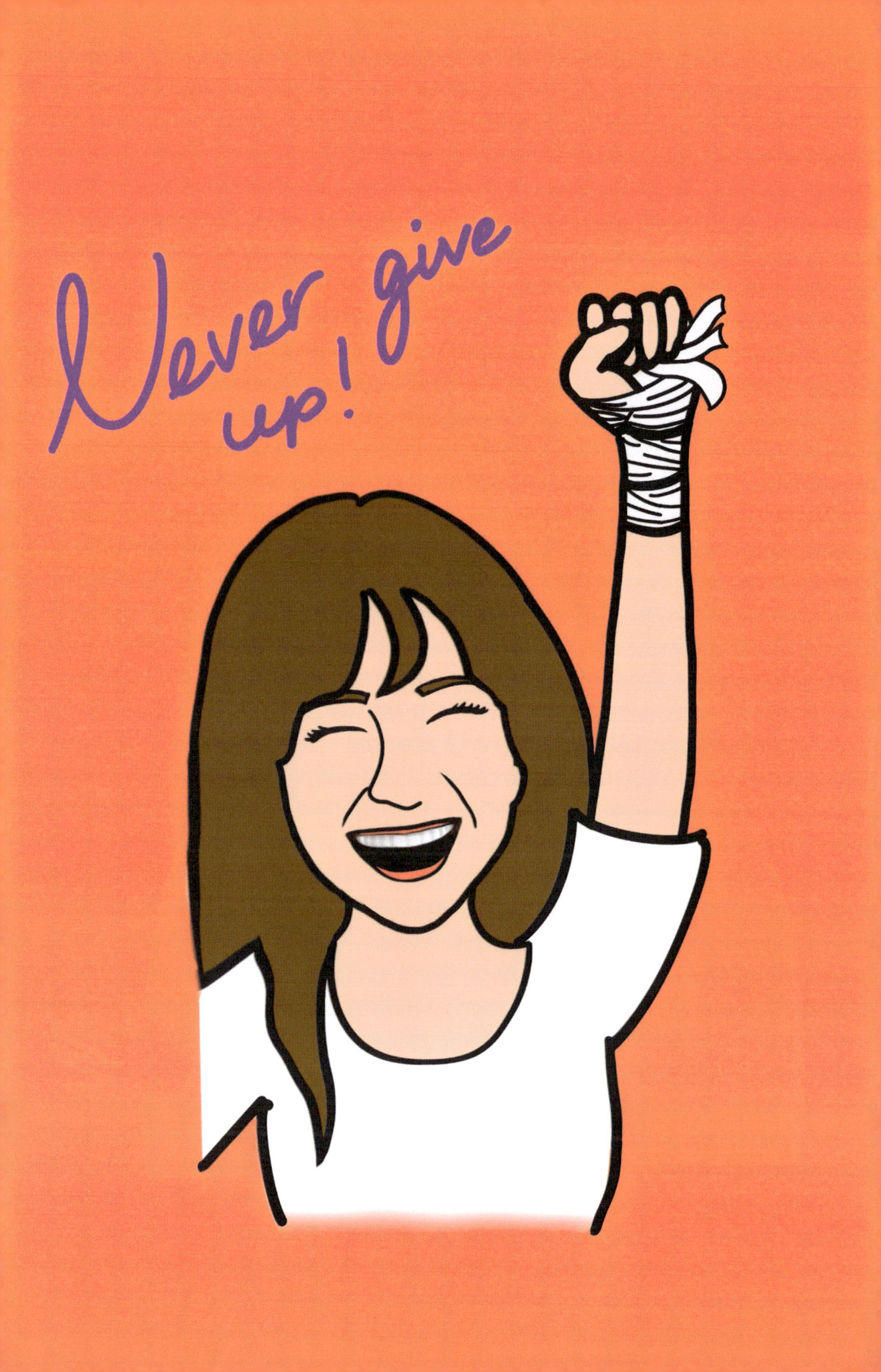

Never give up!

You'll develop more empathy than ever before.

You'll never judge anyone at face value again.

You'll change for the better.

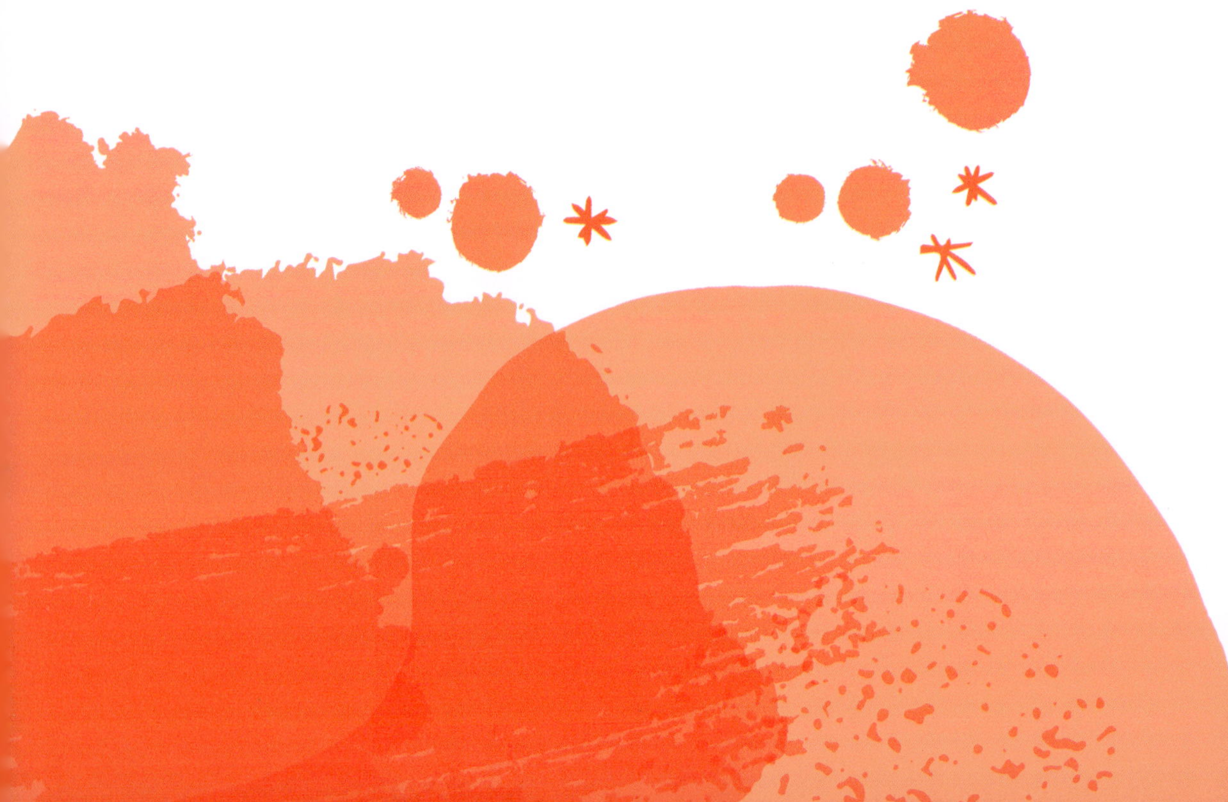

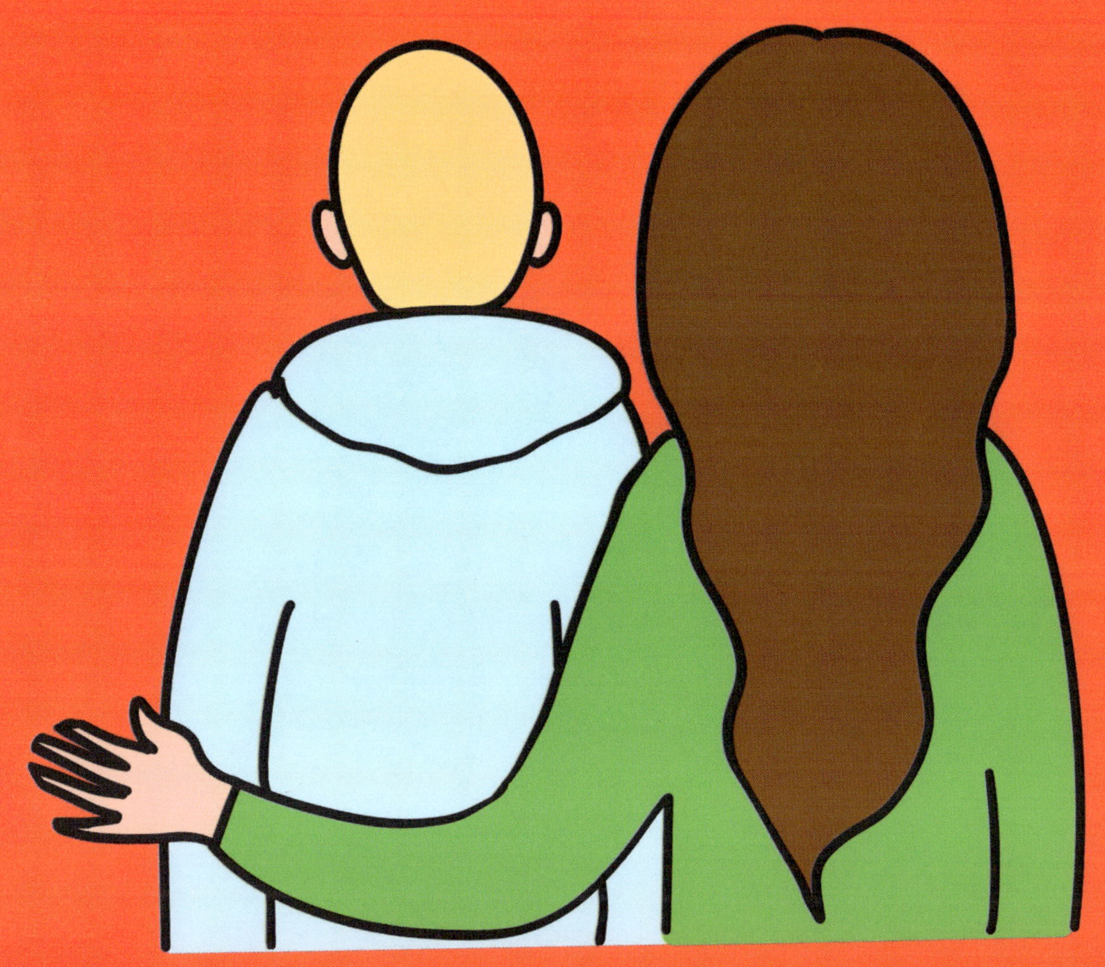

You'll gain true understanding of what is important in life.

Letting go of what doesn't matter.

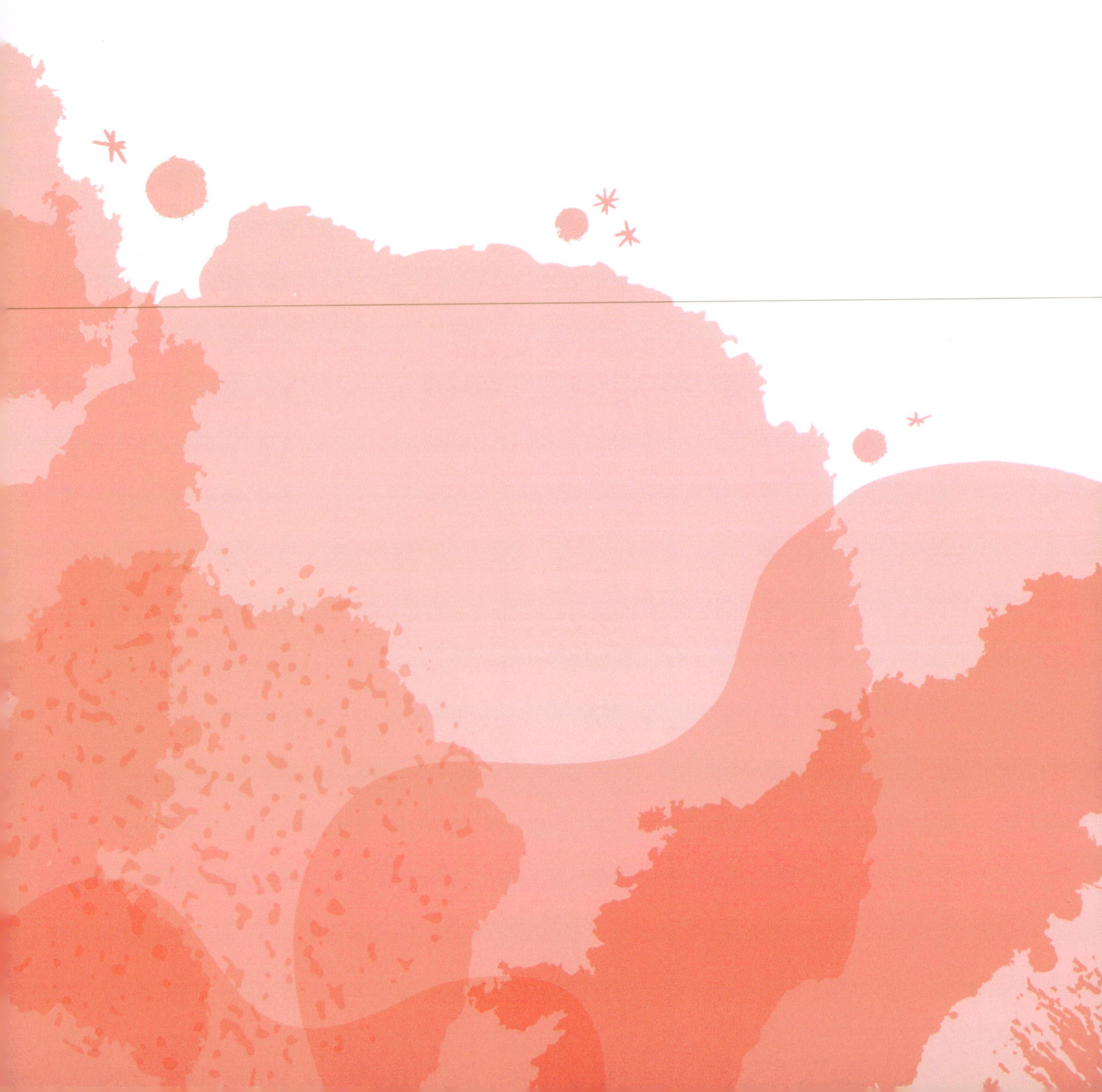

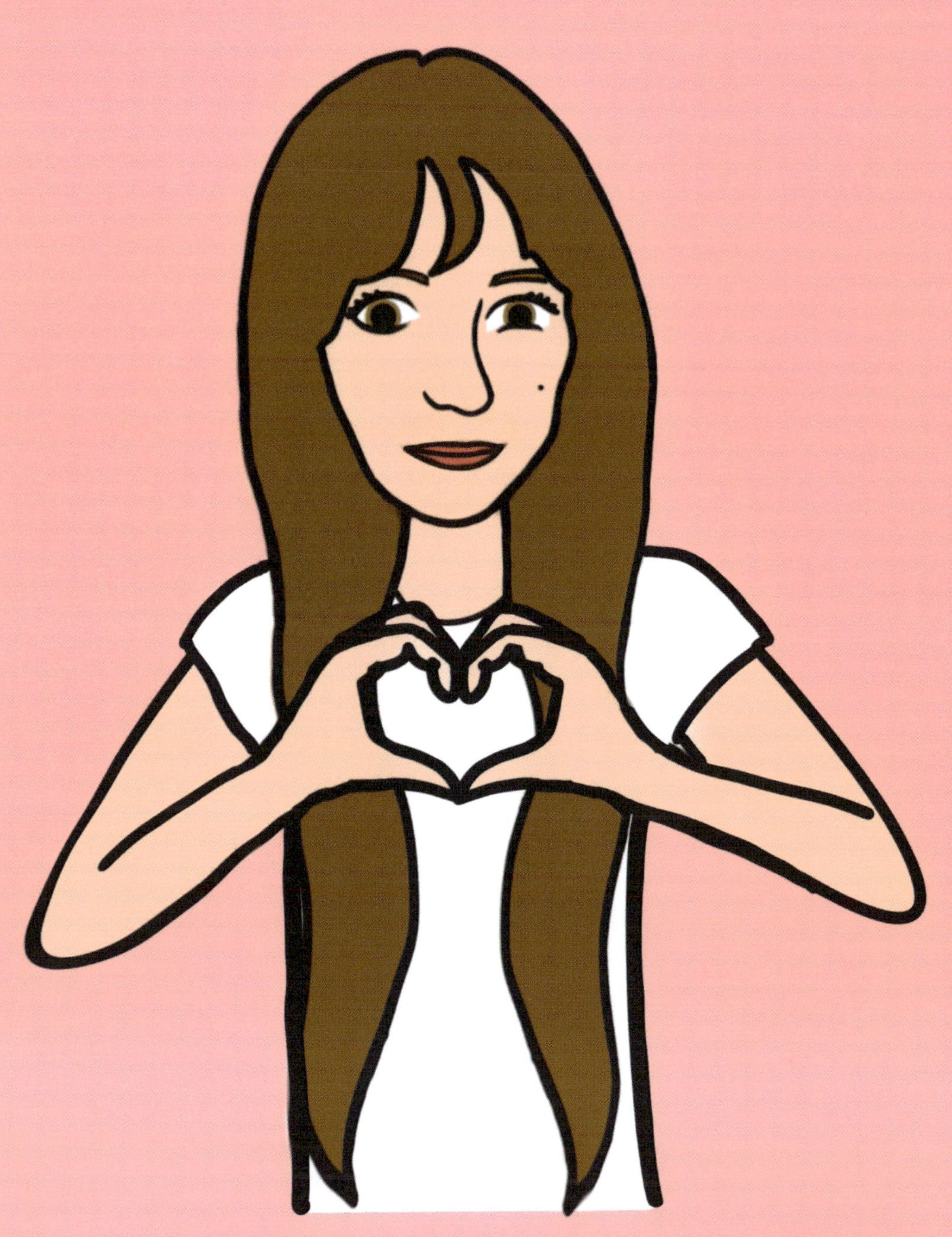

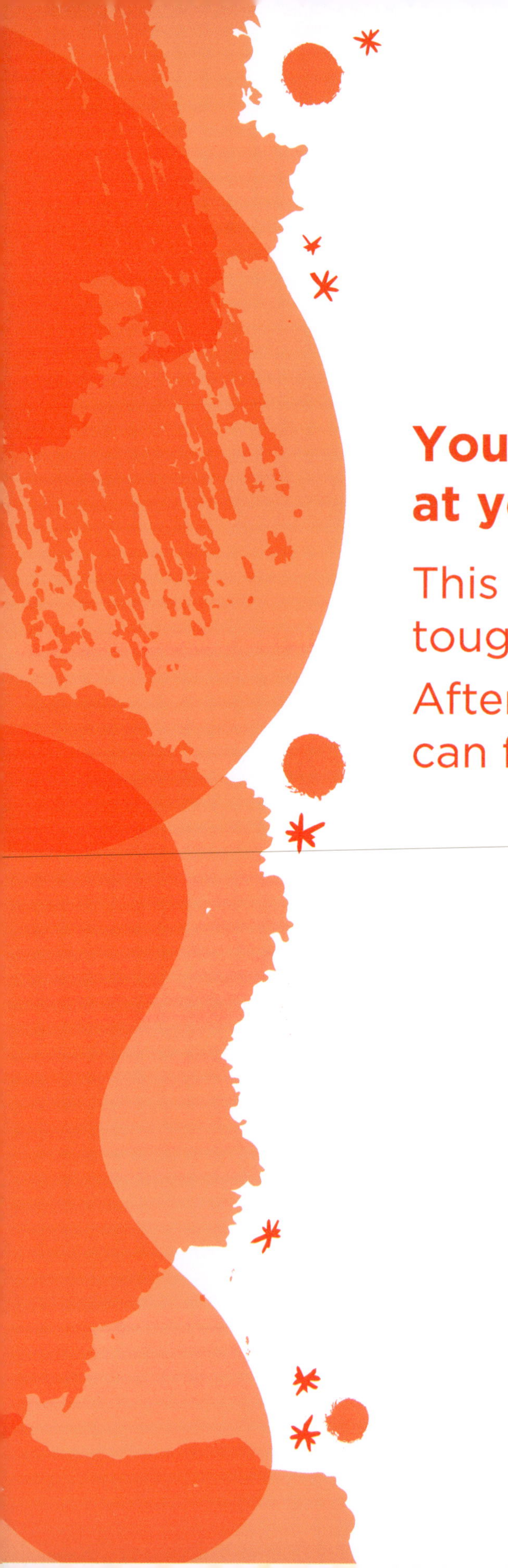

You'll be amazed at your strength.

This will be your toughest journey yet.

After this, you can face anything.

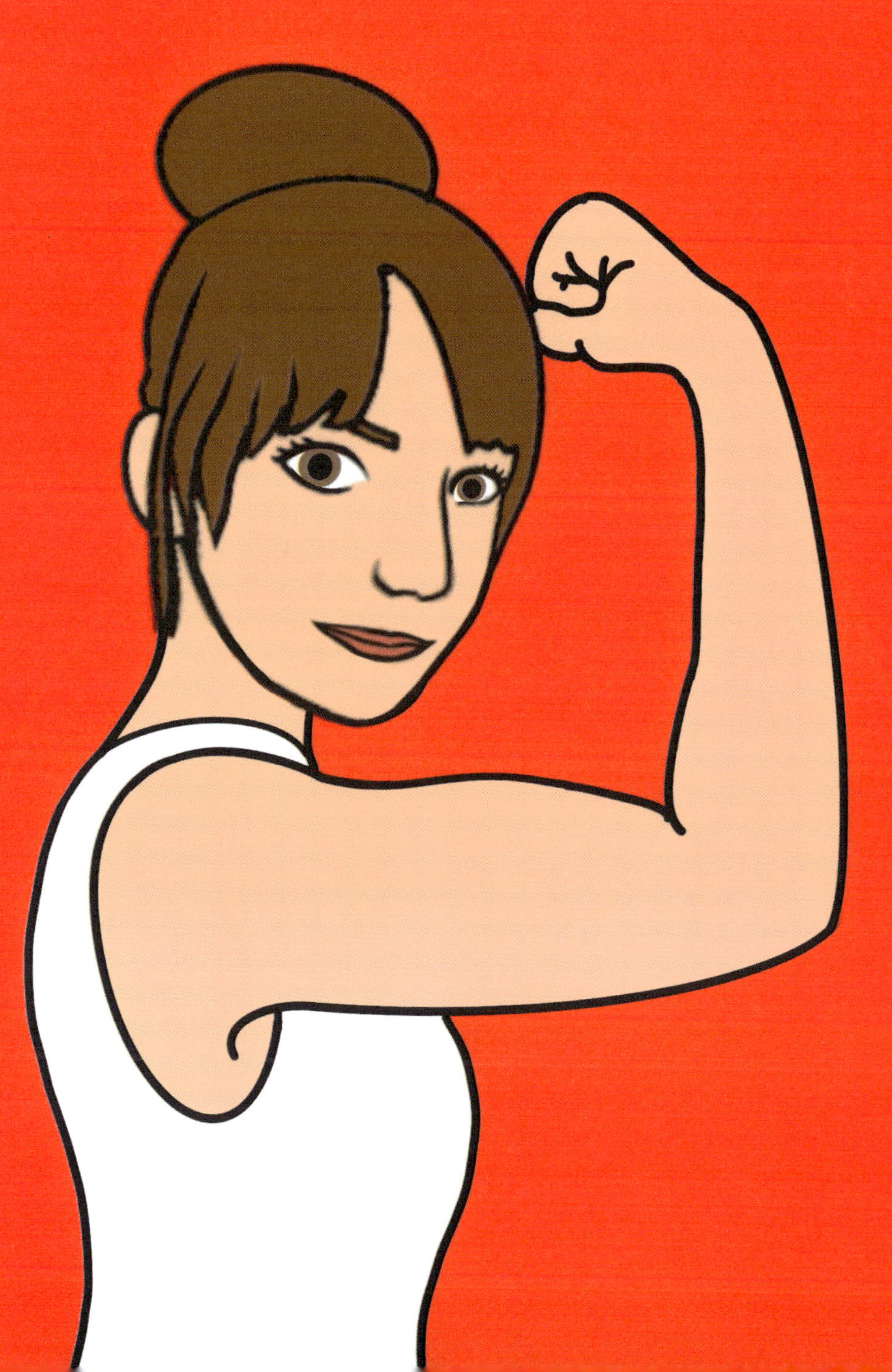

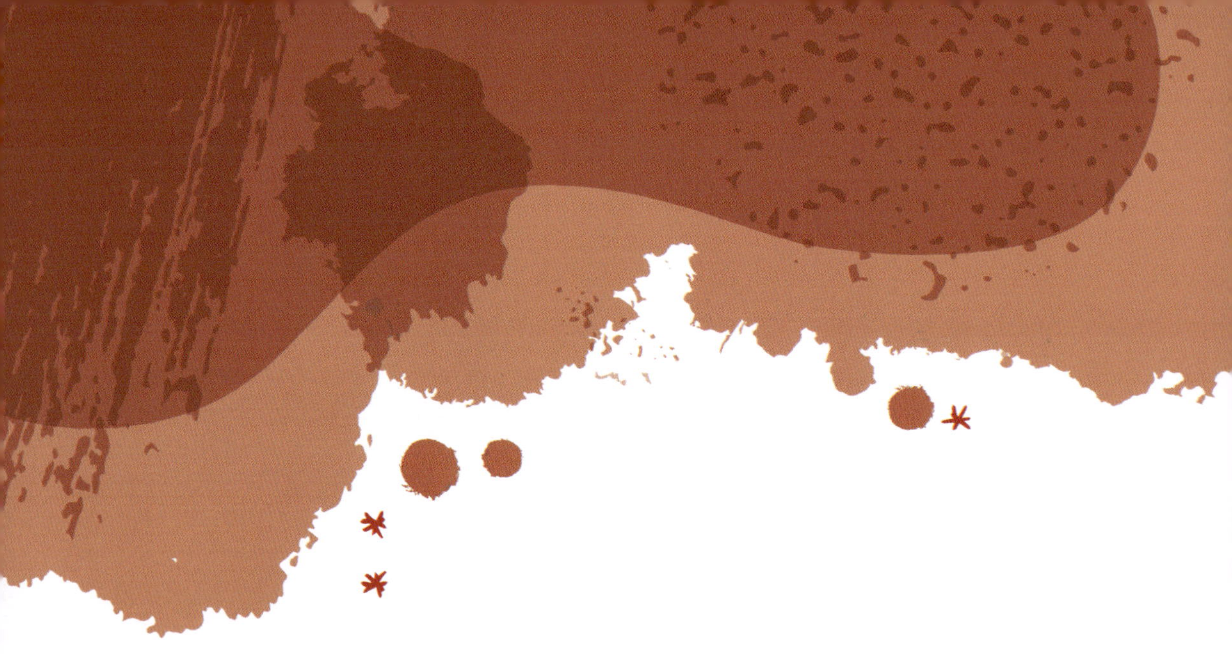

You'll become part of a club you never wanted to belong to.

It will become the most supportive community you could wish for.

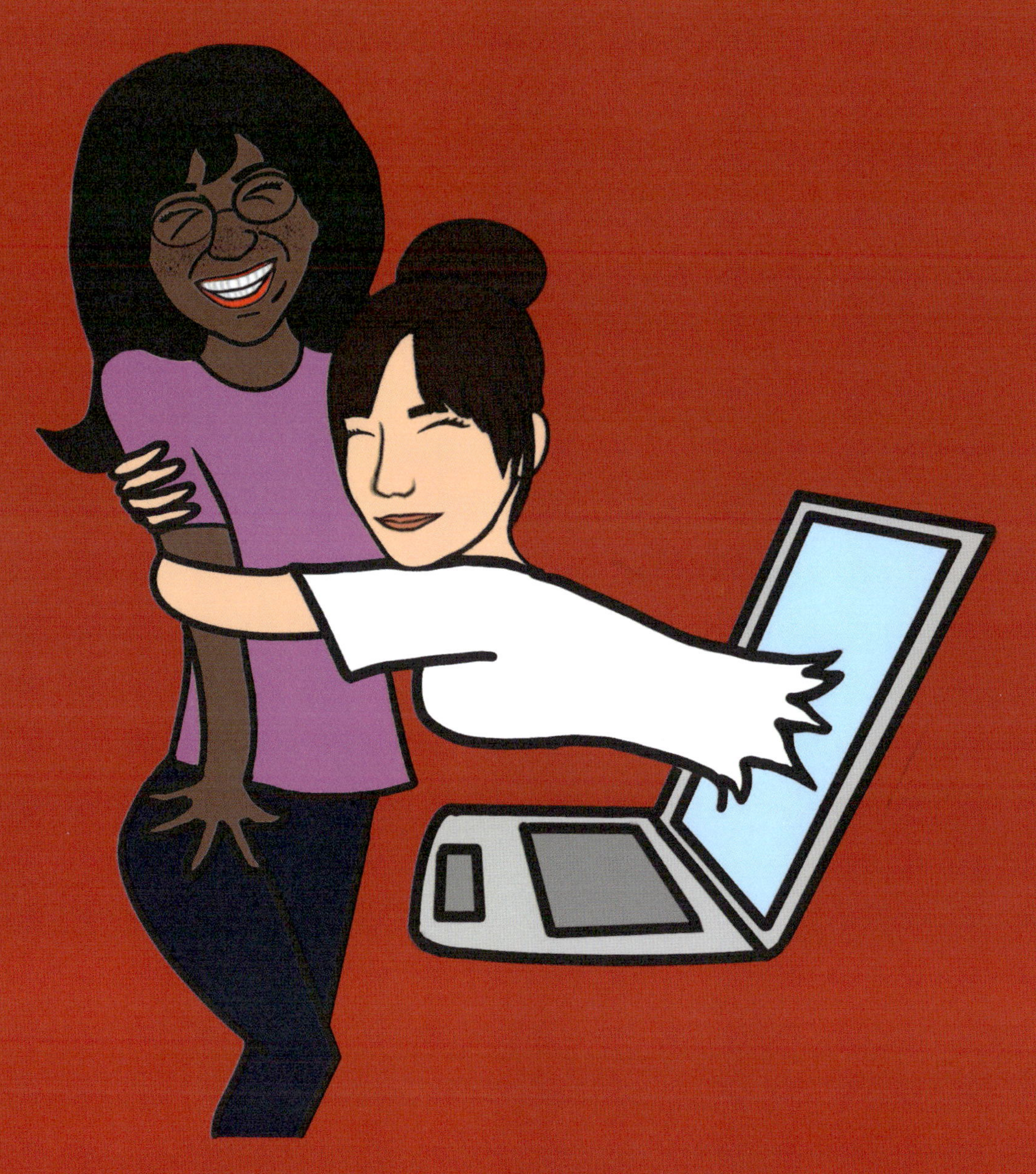

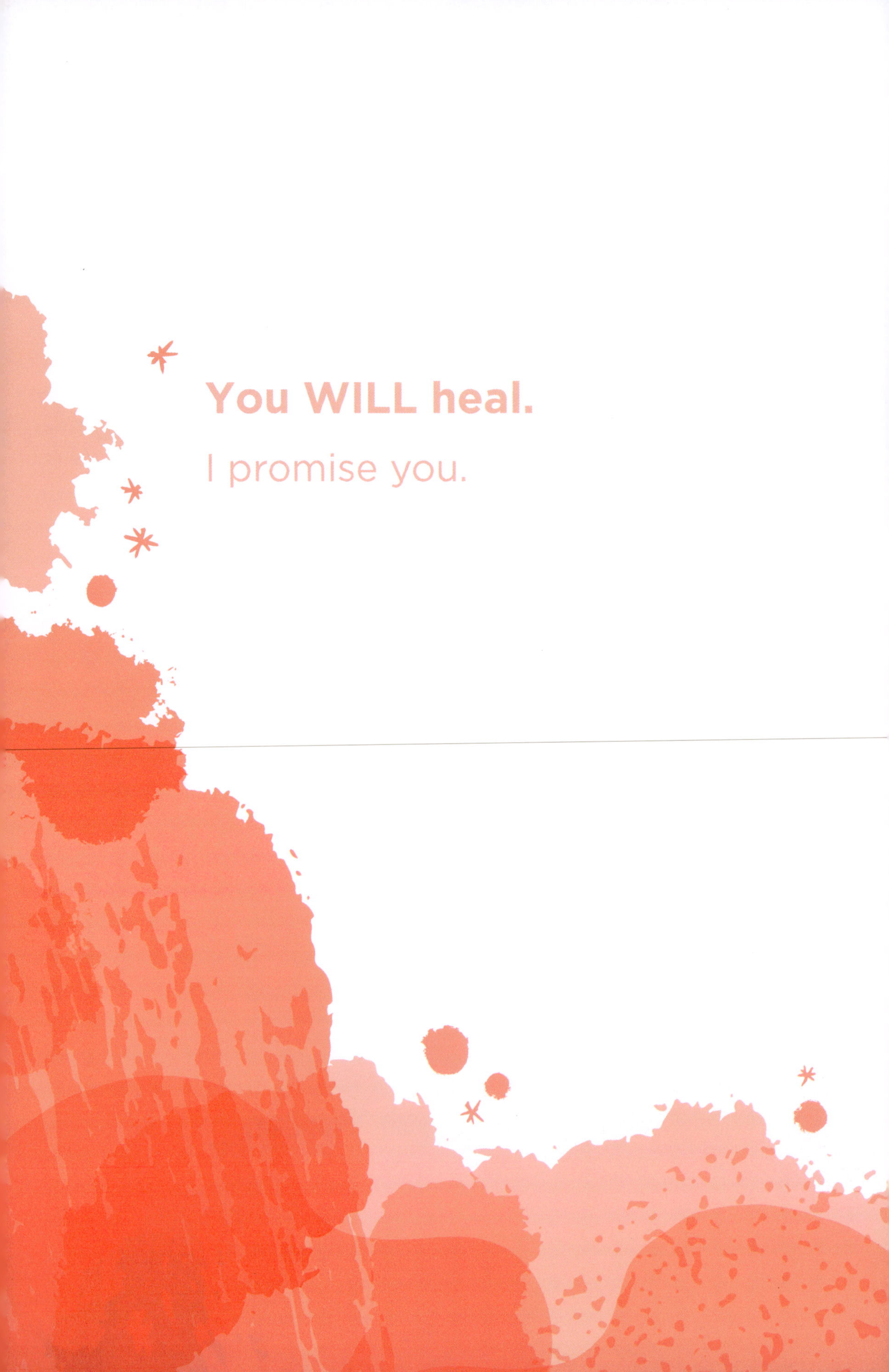

You WILL heal.

I promise you.

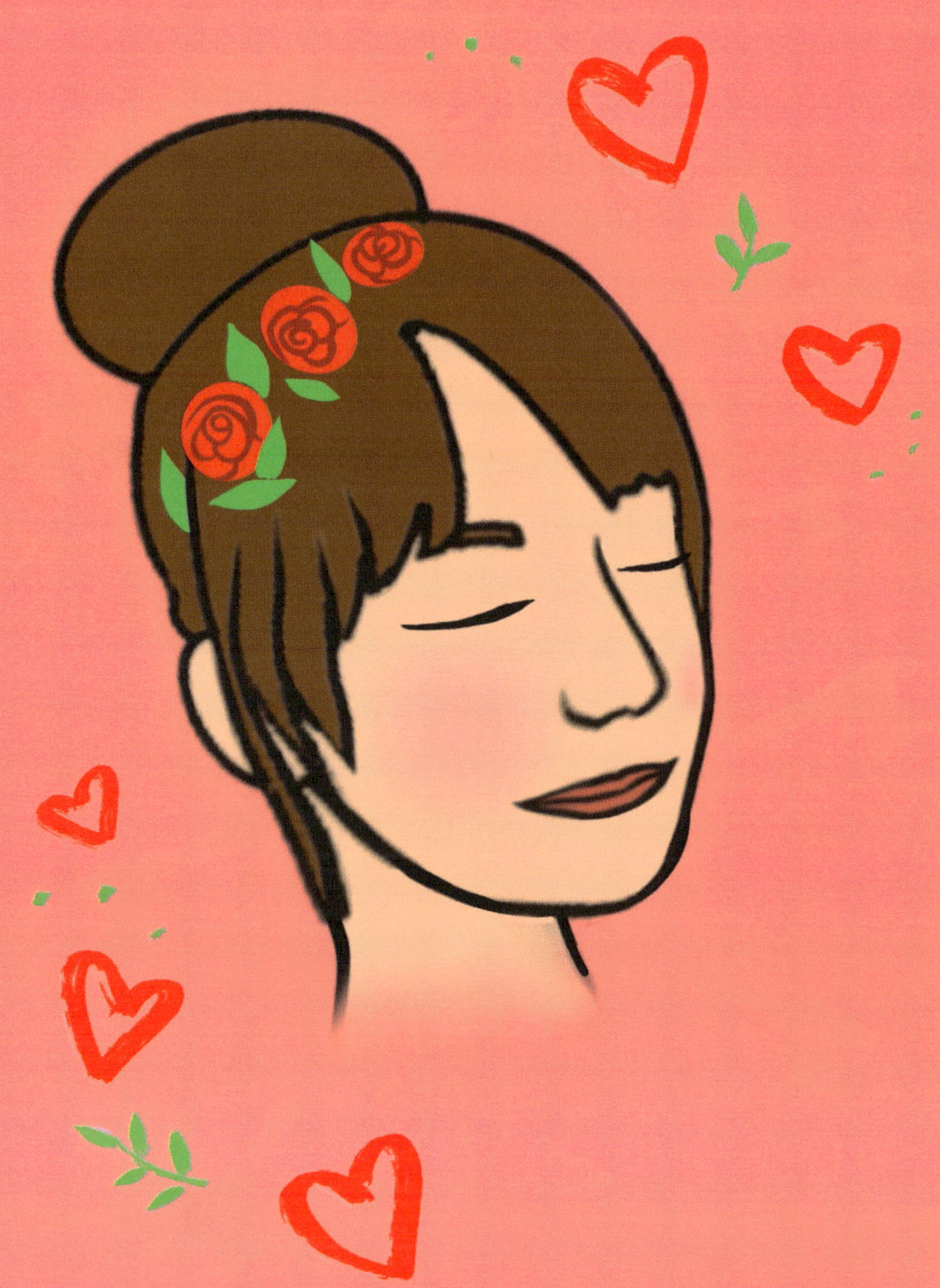

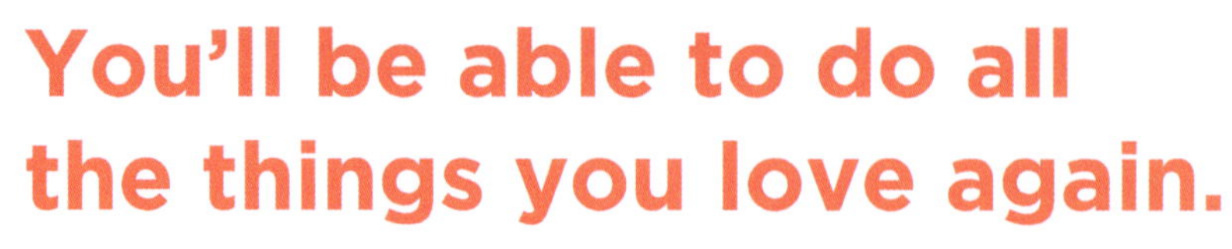

You'll be able to do all the things you love again.

Without worrying about your skin.

Ever.

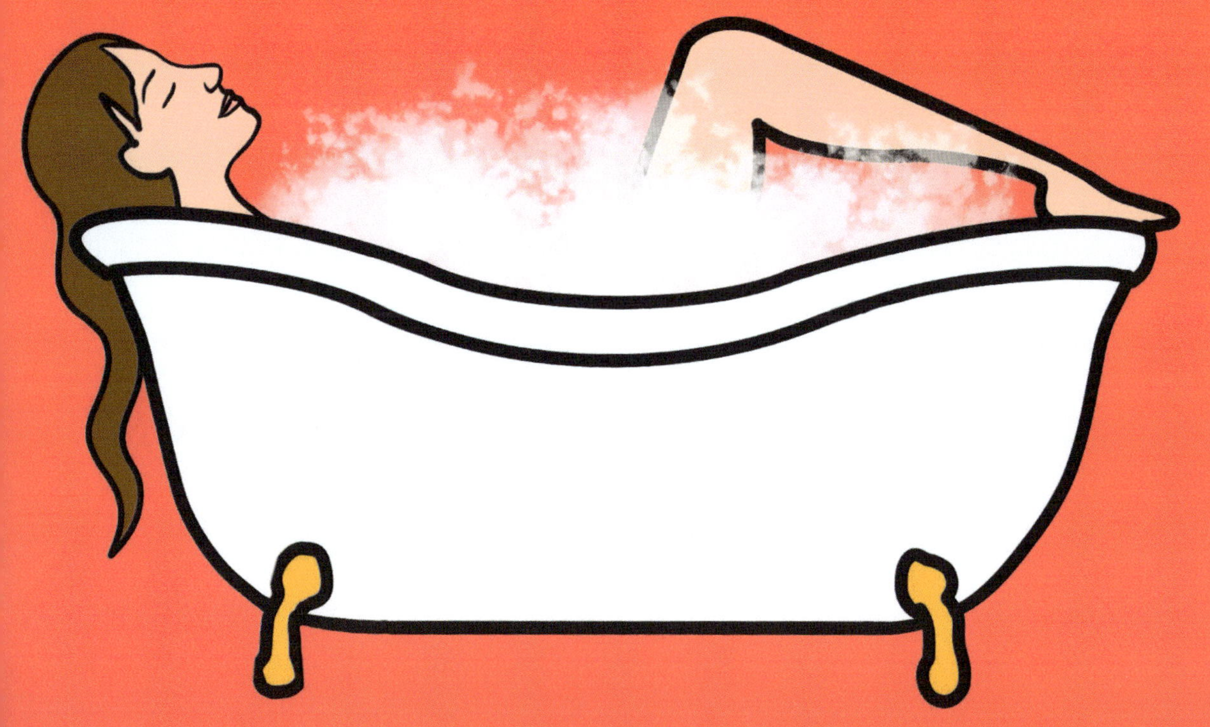

The secret to TSW recovery

At the beginning of my TSW journey, I thought I'd be able to find a way to heal faster than the average recovery time. Ridiculous maybe, but such was my hopefulness.

I thought I'd discover some magical healing technique through my thousands of hours of research and by testing new therapies, vitamins and creams. I thought that surely there was something I could try that no one else had thought of.

Perhaps you, too, are reading this book, hoping I'll spill the secret on what the answer is.

Well, I'm sorry to say, there is no secret formula, no magic pill.

The answer is simply allowing enough time for recovery.

I can understand this is hard to hear when you're in the process of walking through hell. Just know that eventually, your body **will** recover. Unfortunately, it takes time - and a whole lot of patience.

Because it's a form of drug withdrawal, the symptoms can be excruciating. Everyone experiences symptoms to a different extent, in a different order, and on different body parts. In some cases, all symptoms appear; in others, only a few are experienced.

I believe the key to getting through it is to understand that **you will get better** and to make yourself as comfortable as possible throughout each stage or skin flare.

Easing your journey to recovery

This book isn't intended to offer medical advice. However, I thought I'd share some lifestyle changes and alternative treatments that can be effective, based on my own experience. These helped me along the way, and I hope they can help you, too.

Take regular daily exercise

Exercise increases blood flow, which can help the body heal both physically and mentally. I found that any sweat on my body seriously hurt (hello, scratch attack). So instead of pushing myself to that point, I took things more gently. This included lifting a kettlebell or small weights or going for walks each day.

Try a healthy, elimination diet

Not only is healthy eating essential for good health, but the wrong diet can also exacerbate symptoms. Knowing this, I eliminated processed foods, sugar, alcohol and caffeine. I also cut out trigger foods I was sensitive to, such as dairy, wheat, and high salicylate vegetables, fruits, and nuts.

Further into withdrawal, my sensitivities lessened as my body started to heal. At that point, I was able to eat a broader range of foods. I did undergo prick and blood allergy testing. However, my body was so hypersensitive that the results weren't very accurate. Plus, these tests aren't able to identify certain intolerances.

Ultimately, the foods I chose to eliminate were based on my own observed reactions to them.

Give your body the right nutrients

Essential nutrients are vital for good health, and I wanted to ensure my body had everything it needed. It seemed to crave protein and vitamin C, so I started taking supplements to satisfy these 'felt' deficiencies. However, everyone's needs are different.

There are plenty of supplements that may help you or your specific additional needs (such as helping you sleep), but I would advise you to be careful with what you take and to do your research.

Please note: Factors such as diet, supplements and detoxes, won't heal TSW. What I'm trying to get across is that if your body is clearly lacking something or reacting to certain foods, then you need to address it. The last thing you want is for allergens to add to your flares.

Do your best to adopt a healthy mindset

Having a healthy, positive mindset is crucial to recovery success. It's so important to be kind to yourself, and to understand that you're healing and your body is doing an incredible job. Try to keep external stresses to a minimum. Remember that TSW is an itchy condition, and you ARE going to itch. It's impossible not to, so don't feel guilty for scratching.

There's no set timeframe for recovery. Because of this, don't even think about the end. Just try to just get through each day, celebrate the little wins along the way, and don't let the anger or fear consume you. Also, don't become obsessed with recording your progress – and always expect the unexpected.

Healing isn't linear, and neither should you expect your mental mindset to be. Flares will come and go – try to focus on the fact that they will go. I know this is easy for me to say now that I've come out the other side but, believe me, it will get better. The TSW community was my lifeline for guidance, friendship and support during recovery, and they can help you, too.

Give yourself permission to rest

We all know how busy life can be, but make sure you get enough rest. Rest, whether through sleep or relaxation, can play a big part in helping the body heal.

Give yourself permission to slow down and stop as much as possible and accept and ask friends and family for support when you need it. Don't get to the point where your body forces you to rest. Try to rest before you need to.

Cool the discomfort with cryotherapy

Cryotherapy, meaning 'cold therapy', is a technique where the body is exposed to extremely cold temperatures for a certain amount of time.

I only discovered cryotherapy late into my TSW journey, so I can't vouch for its effectiveness early on, but it was a game-changer for me, especially localised cryotherapy on my face. It calmed my sore flaking face considerably.

Try moisture withdrawal treatment

Moisture withdrawal (MW) involves using nothing on the skin. That means no water, creams, moisturisers or lotions. This sounds wrong, but it can work wonders. I did this from the beginning, mainly because everything stung like fire when it touched my skin, so I had no choice. But it was by far the best thing I could have done.

I couldn't shower properly for a year, and, at times, my skin was so flaky I had to do everything in my power not to apply moisturiser. The result, in the end, though, was beyond worth it. My skin eventually began to learn to moisturise itself and healed.

There are people who only feel comfortable lying in bleach baths or in apple cider vinegar, dead sea salt or oils – but for me, these would have been terrible.

Please note: 'No moisture treatment' (NMT) is a step up from MW. You can find information about it online.

Avoid allergens and irritants

The last thing you want is to expose your poor sensitive body to irritants or allergens that could exacerbate a flare.

I avoided strong fragrances, detergents, cleaning products, pollen and grass. I wasn't using any products on my skin as I was doing MW, so I didn't have makeup, moisturisers and the like to worry about.

One thing I would recommend is to vacuum the flakes and dust from your home regularly - they can also worsen symptoms.

Choose soft, breathable materials

Feeling something soft and light against your skin when you have TSW makes clothes more bearable. I lived in shorts and t-shirts (mainly pyjamas) every day for 15 months. Cotton or bamboo clothes have been my go-to. In the early stages, I would wear all my clothes inside out as the seams really hurt my skin.

As well as wearing soft, breathable clothes, I chose equally non-irritating materials for my bedding and towels. I avoided synthetic materials, wool or anything that could make me hot.

Wearing gloves for everything to protect my hands has also been key. Nappy changes, washing up, cutting fruit, wiping the table, you name it. Some people also find bandages and compression clothing works well, especially when oozing.

Put your symptoms on ice

So many TSW sufferers I know are all about the ice ice, baby. And I found ice packs and fans indispensable when it came to minimising flares.

I would always ensure the freezer was full of ice packs, so that I could swap them overnight. I even used ice packs and fans throughout winter; the season didn't make a difference.

Raising hope and awareness

Reflecting on the last 15 months, it's difficult for me to look at my photos and recall my feelings during those darkest days. I still wouldn't say I'm completely healed, but thankfully I'm a world away from the severity of the symptoms I experienced during that first year.

TSW is an iatrogenic condition (it's caused by medical treatment), so it would be untruthful to say that I didn't feel anger for what I've been through. Like many hundreds of thousands of people, I've been made severely ill due to the over-prescription of a medication - something that was 100 per cent avoidable.

It's shocking that TSW and topical steroid addiction were first discussed as early as the 1970s, yet we're still fighting for recognition and awareness. It's even more shocking that potentially millions of people are going through this unknowingly.

People are being diagnosed as having 'severe eczema' and using increasingly potent steroid creams, unaware that what they're using is actually causing their symptoms. They're unwillingly becoming addicted to topical steroids and face years of withdrawal symptoms.

I don't believe that my doctors over the years, in both the UK and Australia, intentionally caused me harm. They genuinely did what they thought best after looking at my skin. However, I now know that medical professionals can only use the knowledge and training they've been given to advise their patients. With such a lack of TSW education and research, it's not surprising this has happened to so many people.

My hope is that we can continue to raise awareness of the potential dangers of topical steroids. To make sure that doctors are better equipped to not only identify TSW but to prevent TSW by ensuring safe steroid use from the start.

As I said at the beginning, not all people who use topical steroids get TSW. It's unknown why certain people are more prone to it. The condition is often referred to as 'rare', but from my own first-hand experience, and after speaking to thousands of people about it, I would argue the opposite.

TSW is not just a skin condition; it's not simply dry skin or an allergic reaction. It's actually nerve damage, oozing, pain, flaking and all of the other symptoms outlined in this book.

Steroids continue to be a vital part of medical treatment. However, my aim is to make sure that the medical professionals prescribing it are aware of the realities and implications of long-term steroid prescriptions.

In the last year alone, I've seen more and more national and international eczema and dermatology organisations recognise and discuss TSW across all forms of media. This is fantastic. With increased awareness and education, overuse of over-prescribed topical steroids should be a thing of the past.

TSW certainly isn't Eczema

There's a wonderful TSW community online that will support you along the way. I've made some amazing friends through all of this, and for that, I'm grateful. You can see more of my own journey @theendlessitch, and I'm here if you ever need an understanding ear.

I've grown so much from having TSW and completely changed as a person. In many ways, it's been both the best and worst thing to happen to me.

Helpful resources

For more information on TSW, please visit the following fantastic resources:

Scratch That: scratchthat.org.uk

Founded in the UK, *Scratch That* is an online information resource, community and awareness campaign for TSW.

This website is an easy to understand informative resource. Their printable 'Condition Card' and 'Appointment Discussion Guide' are valuable assets for anyone with (or associated with) TSW.

ITSAN: itsan.org

The International Topical Steroid Awareness Network is a non profit charity formed to raise awareness about TSW.

The ITSAN site offers a complete comprehensive guide to TSW, with a vast array of resources for both the patient and doctor.

An Overview of TSW (Topical Steroid Withdrawal): youtube.com/watch?v=x4ypA9w81f0

This fantastic Youtube Video by Dr Heba Khaled explores corticosteroid addiction and withdrawal from a medical and patient perspective.

Eczema Association Australia: eczema.org.au

The Eczema Association of Australasia Inc (EAA) was founded with the mission of bringing community support, awareness and mass advocacy to the management and treatment of Eczema.

This offers a brief overview of TSW.

What Allergy: whatallergy.com

What Allergy is a blog run by internationally acclaimed writer and allergy expert, Ruth Holroyd.

Detailing her 2 year battle with TSW, she brings a personal insight into the condition.

Cara Ward Blog: tswcara.blogspot.com

Author of 'Curing my Incurable Eczema', Cara offers hope to all TSW suffers as she outlines her battle through TSW to fully healed.

Preventable: Protecting Our Largest Organ (Full length documentary)

This is available to watch on youtube or the ITSAN website. An incredible documentary by Briana Banos.

Acknowledgements

I'd like to thank my beautiful cousin, Charlotte Oxenham, for all her hard work in creating the fabulous illustrations for this book and for bringing each stage of my journey to life.

Thank you to my friend, Nicole Morris for her wonderful front cover design and creativity.

To Rebecca Dawson who has created such beautiful graphical layouts throughout this whole book and enabled my vision to become reality. Thank you.

Thank you to my loving family for their support throughout.

Last but not least, thank you, dear reader, for helping bring more awareness of topical steroid withdrawal and for welcoming this book into your heart.

Here's to the healing of all TSW warriors.

Printed in Great Britain
by Amazon

56579078R00082